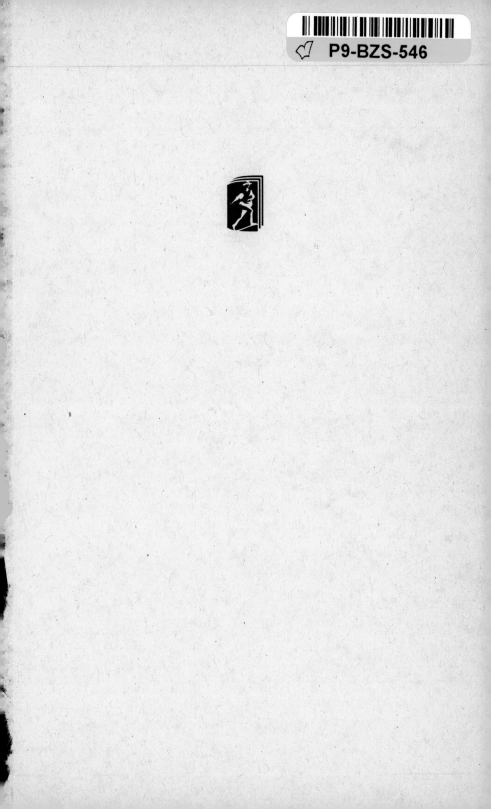

THE
SEX-STARVED
WIFE

What to Do When He's Lost Desire

MICHELE
WEINER DAVIS

SIMON & SCHUSTER PAPERBACKS

NEW YORK LONDON TORONTO SYDNEY

SIMON & SCHUSTER PAPERBACKS
A Division of Simon and Schuster, Inc.
1230 Avenue of the Americas
New York, NY 10020

First Simon & Schuster trade paperback edition January 2009

SIMON & SCHUSTER PAPERBACKS and colophon are registered trademarks of
Simon & Schuster, Inc.

For information regarding special discounts for bulk purchases,
please contact Simon & Schuster Special Sales at
1-800-456-6798 or business@simonandschuster.com.

Designed by Davina Mock

Manufactured in the United States of America

10 8 6 4 2 1 3 5 7 9

The Library of Congress has cataloged the hardcover as follows:
Weiner Davis, Michele.
The sex-starved wife : what to do when he's lost desire / Michele Weiner Davis.
p. cm.
1. Sex in marriage. 2. Sexual desire disorders. I. Title.
HQ734.W43748 2008
613.9'5—dc22
2007042714

ISBN-13: 978-0-7432-6626-0
ISBN-10:   0-7432-6626-9
ISBN-13: 978-0-7432-6627-7 (pbk)
ISBN-10:   0-7432-6627-7 (pbk)

Contents

Acknowledgments

⁓

This book got caught in the birth canal. As John Lennon once said, "Life is what happens when you're busy making plans." In the time I was supposed to be writing, I made a geographical move across the country, both of my children left home, there were family illnesses, my daughter got married, I set up a new business in a new town, and I established myself in a new community with new friends—no small tasks, indeed. Suffice it to say, this book is long overdue. There is no question about who takes top billing on my list of people to appreciate: Sydny Miner, my editor, and her colleagues at Simon & Schuster for patience that has gone far above and beyond the call of duty. Their continued belief in me and support of my work through the past few years has been incredibly touching. In a big bureaucracy like S&S with its many high-maintenance authors, I could have expected to be treated like a number. And that's precisely what happened: I was treated like #1. Thank you for your patience.

As always, my family and friends sustain me in life. My loving and devoted husband, Jim—you've been a constant cheerleader; our two amazing and loving children, Danielle and Zachary; my mother, Elizabeth Weiner; my father, Harry Weiner; plus the newest member of our family, Ryan—I thank you all so much for your love and support. I also want to thank my brothers, Ken and Chuck, and their families for love and caring. My appreciation and love for my mother- and father-in-law, Leah and Bill, has continued throughout the years.

To Virginia Peeples, my dear friend, who is much, much more than my assistant at the Divorce Busting Center: thank you for devoting yourself to making my professional and personal life the best that it can be. My gratitude for your hard work, talent, and dedication is endless.

To Joe Peeples, thank you from the bottom of my heart for so generously sharing your wife and making the Divorce Busting mission possible.

There are other colleagues at my center who enrich my professional life and enable me to be proud of the work we're doing. They include Karen Richards, who has truly become an integral part of our divorce-busting mission—I can't imagine what we'd do without her. That's also true for Joann Sallmann, Vernetta Mickey, Laurie Chaplin, Chuck Fallon, Dotty Decker, Jody Stratford, Susie Ryder, Jerry Schreur, Claudia Murphy, and Mark McGunnigle. Thanks for being such an incredible team and for the work you do to help couples restore their love.

I have also relied on other colleagues for support, insight, or assistance with the manuscript, and they have given of their time generously: Michael Yapko, my friend and wise adviser; Tina Pittman, friend and research brainstormer, Barry McCarthy the academic voice of reason; and Diane Sollee, my fan and cheerleader. Other colleagues on my thank-you list are Pat Love, Stephen Stosny, Bill O'Hanlon, Jeff Zeig, and Rich Simon. Special thanks to Jeannie Kim for her help with the *Redbook* Sex Survey. Special thanks too to Mary Kelly-Williams for her enormous help with the resources chapter.

My appreciation goes to Suzanne Gluck, my long-time agent, for her continued belief in my writing.

And then there are my friends, both old and new, who deeply enrich my life: Noble Golden, Sharon Chewning, Therese Quoss, Arnold Woodruff, Diane Israel, Mary Kelly-Williams, Anita Koury, Claudia Murphy, Susie Ryder, and Susan Mann.

Last, but certainly not least, are the many women who were brave enough to share their lives and stories with me and to entrust me to help them create more love, lust, and laughter in their lives. Thank you for teaching me so much about this very important topic: the sex-starved wife.

This book is dedicated to close friends and family who have surfed the waves with me over the last few years. Thank you all.

Introduction

New love is the brightest, and long love is the greatest,
but revived love is the tenderest thing known on earth.
                                                    —Thomas Hardy

Are you a sex-starved wife? A woman who deeply desires more satisfying sex with your husband? Would you settle for just *more* sex? Or to put it more accurately, would *some* sex do? If so, I am not surprised that the title of this book piqued your interest. You are craving a loving, passionate, juicy, sexual relationship with your man. And you deserve it! The good news is that you've come to the right place. Although we've never met, I know what you've been going through and how the difference in your and your husband's sex drives has taken a toll on you. I also know that until now, effective help for your problem has been in short supply. But that's all about to change. I am going to be your personal coach and help you become an expert on getting your love life back on track.

But first, I want you to read a few letters from women who have been struggling with a desire gap in their own marriages. You're about to learn that you, my friend, are not alone:

Hi Michele,

My husband is just not interested in sex. He has no desire for me. Unless we go away and stay at a hotel or it is a special occasion, he will do anything to avoid the sex. When we do have sex, he won't touch certain parts of my body. He won't kiss. He won't say, "I love you" either. I feel worthless, ugly, undeserving. I am obsessed by the lack of sex in our relationship. When I bring it up, he gets angry and says that he should just leave, that all I want to do is create drama where there is none. Most days I just wish I could run away and not feel anymore. I am dying inside and don't know how much longer I can hang on.

———————————

Dear Michele,

My husband's libido has been at rock bottom for years. Always believing it would get better, I've stuck it out. But now I feel I am losing the best years of my life, as well as my libido. Am I not allowed to feel feminine? We have sex three to four times a year; he orgasms upon penetration, leaving me wanting more than a "clean-up" job and a good, silent cry in the bathroom. He knows I'm upset. He is laissez-faire about seeking help.

I am attractive. I am very lonely with my children grown. I desperately need to feel the arms of a loving man around me once again. My husband's attempts are robotic, in an effort to keep me from divorcing him. Where am I in his emotional absence? Where am I in his life? I'd give my eyes and teeth for good sex once a year!

Does any of this sound familiar? Are you longing for more touch, sex, and physical closeness? Are you overwhelmed by feelings of hurt, rejection, loneliness, and frustration? Do you find yourself wondering what's wrong with you because your husband doesn't seem interested? Have you been so desperate that you've even considered (or are) having an affair? Do you feel ashamed that your husband isn't like other men? Have you grown increasingly exasperated that you haven't been able to get your husband to understand what's missing in your relationship? If so, hear this—there are millions of women out there who, contrary to popular belief, feel *exactly* the same way you do.

Perhaps you're wondering where all these women live, because all you ever hear about are horny husbands with nearly permanent erections who chase their wives around the dining room table. Your friends at your health club complain that their husbands' sexual needs are moving targets: the more sex they get, the more they want. They can't stand their husbands' need for constant physical reassurance. And think about the

media. Hardly a day passes without some magazine or newspaper article, medical study, or relationship expert offering women advice for stoking their sexual flames and rekindling their desire. The message is clear: men have insatiable sexual appetites; women have headaches.

And then there's your marriage.

Perhaps it started out on fire; you couldn't keep your hands off each other, and your lovemaking was frequent and passionate. But somewhere along the line, things changed. Maybe it was when you got pregnant or when the kids were born. Or perhaps the problem started when his job became ultrastressful. It might have been around the time you started arguing about money, in-laws, or who does what around the house. Maybe it was the twenty pounds you gained or the medicine he takes every day. Or his lack of interest in sex could have something to do with his difficulties maintaining an erection, you wonder. You got dizzy trying to figure things out.

Maybe the signs of your husband's sexual sluggishness were there all along. Looking back, you now realize that you just assumed things would get better. But time passed and nothing changed. In fact, things even got worse. He almost never seems interested in you. So, out of desperation, you resigned yourself to the role of initiator. You had to. If it weren't for you, in fact, you'd never have sex. But now you've grown tired of always being the one to reach out, always being the one to risk rejection, always being the one who cares. And the fights about sex have become exasperating. The loneliness is slowly killing you. And he just doesn't get it. Or, you wonder, "Worse yet, does he? Is he doing this to punish me?"

Finally, when analyzing your feelings, his feelings, your marriage, your motives, his intentions, has gotten you nowhere, perhaps you have tried to get your husband to do something about his lack of desire—talk to your family doctor, get a checkup, go to a therapist. But he won't. He can't understand why you're making such a big deal about this sex thing and why you simply won't stop nagging. Everything would be okay, he tells you, if you would just back off.

Or maybe he has gotten medical or psychological advice in the past but his follow-through stinks. You've grown weary of repeating, "What good does testosterone do sitting on a nightstand?" You don't want to pressure him and damage his fragile male ego. You just don't know what to do anymore.

How can you openly admit that the man you married, the man you love, the man with whom you plan on spending the rest of your life, doesn't desire you? You ask yourself, "What's wrong with me. Aren't I attractive?" How did you manage to hook up with the one man in the world who would prefer doing just about anything other than making love to you? Why isn't he like all the other guys?

Well your husband may not be like all the other guys, but you're about to discover that he isn't as unique as you think. In fact, after almost three decades of working with couples and knowing what really goes on behind closed doors, I'm here to tell you that your guy isn't unique at all. Believe it or not, there are millions of men who, for a variety of reasons, just aren't in the mood. In fact, I'm convinced that low sexual desire in men is America's best-kept secret. But why, you ask yourself, should this topic be so hush-hush when women talk openly about their "Not tonight, dear" declarations with anyone who will listen? The short answer: it's different for men.

A woman is expected to have dips in her desire for sex; she can talk about it without her femininity or sanity being called into question. A woman can commiserate with her friends about her husband's one-track mind and how she can't hug him without his thinking sex is imminent and be in really good company. (As one man in my practice put it when I tried to normalize his wife's low desire by saying that she's in good company, he said, "I wouldn't say she's 'in good company.' I'd say she has lots of company.")

Because in our culture masculinity and virility are inextricably connected, most men don't share that level of comfort with self-disclosure. In fact, it strikes terror in their hearts to even think that they don't desire sex, let alone admit it publicly.

Imagine a guy sitting around with his male buddies in the locker room saying, "I just hate my wife's one-track mind. All she ever thinks about is sex. I can't even lie next to her in bed without her starting to grope me. I wish she would be interested in me as a person and not just interested in my body." It doesn't happen.

What's the fallout of all this? To begin with, I feel certain that the incidence of low desire in men is vastly underreported. Why? There's too much shame and embarrassment. And that's a tragedy. If men don't talk to their wives, their friends, or their doctors, why in the world would they talk openly to researchers? They probably don't! And because we don't have accurate statistics, men who lack desire believe they are in a very small minority. Feeling like freaks of nature, they remain isolated and don't get the help they need. As a result, their self-esteem and their marriages suffer.

Secondly, since men don't talk about this, their wives wonder what's wrong with *them*. They believe they're flawed or unattractive. They've had nowhere to turn. Until now.

I have been a marriage therapist for almost three decades, specializing in marriages that other therapists declare dead on arrival. To me, there is no such thing as a marriage that can't be resuscitated. Although helping couples on the brink of divorce is challenging work, I wouldn't trade what I do for anything else. I see miracles happen every day: couples who truly believe divorce is inevitable gradually discover that with a little information, a lot of coaching, and a willingness to leave blame behind, they can reinvent their marriages.

Some years ago, I noticed that many couples in my practice were experiencing major relationship breakdowns because their levels of interest in sex were worlds apart. One spouse was hot, while the other was not. While this sort of disparity happens from time to time in even the best of relationships, there was nothing temporary about the sexual divide wreaking havoc in these marriages. There were long-standing issues of rejection and misunderstanding that spilled over into every aspect of the couples' lives together. I called these relationships *sex-starved marriages*.

Contrary to what you might think, a sex-starved marriage is not necessarily one that has no sex (although abstinence can and does occur); it is a marriage where one spouse desperately longs for more touch, physical connection and sex, while the other spouse, for a variety of reasons, just isn't interested. The partner with lower desire can't understand why his or her spouse seems so obsessed with their sexual relationship and thinks, "What's the big deal? It's just sex."

However, to the spouse with a higher sexual drive—in this case, you (for the sake of simplicity, let's refer to you as the HDS—higher-drive spouse)—it's a huge deal, and it's not just about sex. It's about feeling wanted, loved, appreciated, sexy, and attractive. It's about feeling close and connected. Sex is truly the tie that binds; it leads to emotional intimacy.

And when the spouse with a lower sex drive doesn't understand this, it spells trouble for the marriage.

Longing for more physical closeness, the HDS tries to get his or her partner, the LDS (lower-drive spouse), to understand the importance of having a good sexual relationship. Since she or he doesn't feel the same way, the words fall on deaf ears, and as a result, nothing changes. So the HDS tries again to get through to his or her spouse. Now the LDS feels pressured, angry, and resentful. At this point, intimacy on all levels drops out of the marriage. The spouses stop sitting next to each other on the couch. They stop laughing at each other's jokes. They stop making eye contact. Their talk is perfunctory. They quit being friends. Their marriage is placed at risk of infidelity or divorce.

I found these marriages were so prevalent that I decided to write a book on the subject and called it—you guessed it—*The Sex-Starved Marriage*. I wrote about the problems that occur in marriage when one spouse is vastly more interested in sex than the other and, more important, what they could do to fix things.

The Sex-Starved Marriage was written for both the HDS and the LDS, to help them understand each other's feelings and offer a game plan for taking their sex life off the back burner and making it more of a priority. Among many other things, I was outspoken about the value of a robust sex life for *both* spouses, not just the HDS.

It was in that book that I also spilled the beans: women don't have a corner on the low desire market. Based on my observations in my clinical practice with couples, I knew that many men just weren't in the mood for sex. I felt certain that we as a society have perpetuated a myth about the ever-turned-on male. During my travels on the seminar circuit, I have spoken to countless sex and marital therapists across the country and asked them about their observations about low-desire men. They all agreed that although more men than women complain of not having enough sex, the differences between genders aren't as great as we've been led to believe. Only when we realize how commonplace low desire in men really is will women stop feeling unattractive and come out of hiding to seek the help they need to have richer and more satisfying sexual relationships. That's why I'm so passionate about getting the word out that men have "headaches" too.

Soon after the publication of *The Sex-Starved Marriage*, I was flooded with letters, e-mails and phone calls from people from all walks of life. There were expressions of gratitude from more highly sexed spouses for my having taken a strong stand about the importance of sexuality in marriage and for gently but firmly nudging spouses with a lower sex drive to take a more active role in bridging the desire gap, along with countless requests for more information and marital help. Most striking, however, was the overwhelming reaction from women like you whose husbands have lost desire.

Michele,

I just recently found your book *The Sex-Starved Marriage* in a local bookstore, opened the book, and began to read. My heart began to thump and beat quickly while tears fell from my face. By the time I struck up the nerve to purchase the book, I had already read 60% of it. You see, it is very rare (as you know) for women to talk about the lack of sex in their marriages. It would be wonderful to have more focus on this "role reversal" so that men with low sexual desire are not ashamed. Plus, I need more help! My husband and I are "stuck." We seem unable to find that perfect time to talk. We have been married for fifteen years this August, with two children ages eleven & almost nine. We are high school sweethearts, and I believe we are meant to be together forever; however, I can't go on this way. Can you help?

Sincerely,
"I miss sex with my husband"

Michele,

Oh, my God! I watched you on the *20/20* show, and I cried all the way through it. I wish that my husband could have watched it with me so that he would know how I am feeling. I feel like we never have sex. It has been almost four months, but he doesn't have a clue that it has been that long. We have been married for fifteen years and have three children. We both work full-time jobs, and he is able to find time for everything and everyone but me. I told him the other day that I feel as if he doesn't love me. We hardly ever touch or kiss. I am just overwhelmed after seeing the show that I am not the only wife crying herself to sleep at night because of rejection from my husband.

Michele,

I should like to thank you for addressing such a sensitive subject on prime time television. My husband and I have been together for nearly thirty years and we have five beautiful children. He is thirteen years older than I am. He used to be very sexually active, but in the last ten years it just abruptly stopped. I cannot tell you how lonely it can be. I just wanted to personally thank you so much for opening the door and making me realize that I am not alone.

Something else interesting happened: during the promotion of *The Sex-Starved Marriage*, I was interviewed on countless call-in radio shows. Guess who called in. HD men called to complain about their unsatisfying sex lives. LD women wondered what they could do to increase their sexual desire or to get their husbands to better understand their feelings. Grateful HD women called to thank me for letting them know they're not alone and to discuss their frustration about their husband's apparent lack of empathy. But conspicuously absent were LD men. Not a single man who was lacking sexual desire called in for information or to simply discuss his feelings. Although these phone calls were anonymous, no LD man felt safe talking about this taboo subject. Even when the shows' hosts specifically invited these men to call in, there were no calls. I knew something had to change. As long as the topic of low sexual desire in men is off-limits, women's pain and shame will also remain largely unaddressed. And that's not okay.

Furthermore, it became increasingly obvious to me that even when women were willing to risk talking about their situations, there was precious little effective help available to them. Although *The Sex-Starved Marriage* offered guidance and reassurance, it is largely unisex in its approach and left more highly sexed women with many unanswered questions. And while some of the experiences, emotions, and strategies for overcoming a sexual divide are similar in all marriages regardless of gender, apparently not all are. Sex-starved women face unique challenges, requiring more guidance and support.

So you now know the genesis of this book. What you don't know is what you'll learn by reading it. Maybe for the first time in your marriage, you will see that all the emotions you've been feeling are both understandable and normal. You will learn about what really goes on behind closed doors in bedrooms across America, and you might be very surprised, you will recognize that you are in very good company. You'll start feeling better about yourself as a person and as a sexual being, your festering insecurities caused by the dynamics of your interactions around sex will be replaced by feelings of confidence and empowerment. But this isn't just a feel-good book. By the time you've finished reading it, you'll know more about low desire in men, what causes it, and what you can do to motivate your husband to become more proactive in boosting his desire. You'll have a game plan. You'll stop thinking about divorce or fantasizing about having an affair. And if you've gone outside your marriage to satisfy your sexual needs, you will probably rethink your actions and reinvest yourself in your marriage. That's because at bottom, you really know that you want your spouse, not someone else, to want you.

The Sex-Starved Wife will also answer questions that many women in similar situations to yours have asked me. Although men experience low sexual desire for a variety of reasons, sexual difficulties are one of the most common causes. Almost 30 percent of men have persistent problems with climaxing too early or have difficulty achieving erections. It's easy to understand why a man would avoid sex if he associates it with failure. I will offer you information that will help you approach your husband sensitively, making it more likely that he will be willing to get help for this very solvable problem.

Or perhaps you feel certain that sexual desire isn't the problem; the problem has to do with his lack of desire for *you*. He may be involved with pornography—both online and offline—and you simply can't fathom why he would be masturbating rather than making love to you. You want to know how to get your husband to stop putting energy into his self-interests and focus on you and your marriage. *The Sex-Starved Wife* offers answers to these problems and provides a fascinating look into this growing problem in our society: Internet sex and self-sex as a substitute for marital sex.

In Chapter 1, you will read the surprising results of a poll conducted by *Redbook* magazine and myself. We teamed up to find out what women have to say about their sexual appetites, their husbands' sex drive, and their sexual relationships. Once you and your husband have the facts at your fingertips, you will be armed with information that will be freeing. It will enable you to approach your sexual desire gap more openly and more collaboratively.

Chapter 2 will help you see why your feelings of shame, anger, hurt, and resentment have made reaching out for help so difficult. It is here that you will learn ways to stop blaming yourself (or your spouse) for your less-than-satisfying sexual relationship and start getting ready to create major changes in your life.

In Part II, "Why Men Say No," you'll read about the many explanations for low desire in men. Chapter 3 will help you understand how hormone deficiencies or sexual dysfunctions might be causing your husband's dip in desire. Chapter 4 explores how issues such as depression, stress, or poor body image may be at the root of this problem. And in Chapter 5, you'll learn that common relationship problems such as resentment or anger may be the desire busters. You'll also read about the ways in which pornography, masturbation, and infidelity might be the cause of your sexual distance.

Now that you know about the reasons there is a desire gap in your relationship, it's time to do something about it. And that's what Part III is all about that.

In Chapter 6, you will find new ideas about how best to approach your man. Perhaps you haven't wanted to hurt him, or more likely, you've talked until the cows came home, and the only responses you've gotten are defensiveness and anger. Let's face it: you're dealing with a fragile male ego, so I'll show you how to say and do things that will allow him to keep an open mind and heart.

Chapter 7 describes treatments for helping your husband overcome a drop in desire stemming from biological issues or sexual dysfunction. You will learn ways to approach your husband to get him to go to your family doctor or a marital or sex therapist and the best way to encourage your

husband to follow through on suggestions from his health care profes-sionals. You'll find strategies couples can use together to solve their sexual problems as a team.

In Chapter 8, you will learn ways to help your husband cope with and overcome such problems as depression, poor body image, unresolved childhood issues, grief, job loss, and stress, which may be dampening his desire. While you can't resolve your man's problems for him, there are things you can do to pave the road for his feeling better—and therefore more sexual.

Show me a couple with a desire gap, and I will show you a couple with relationship challenges. In Chapter 9, you will learn how to tackle these problems in loving, effective ways. You will also read about specific tech-niques for being more open about sex and resolving your sexual differ-ences.

Getting one's sexual relationship on track is one thing, but keeping it that way is quite another. Chapter 10 will help you sustain the changes you're making in your love life. This chapter outlines some of the major challenges to keeping passion alive in a marriage, especially when differ-ences have divided couples. It sets out specific steps in order to resist taking positive changes for granted.

Chapter 11 is designed especially for the woman whose husband has stubbornly defied her efforts to make their sexual relationship more sat-isfying. Sometimes, despite a woman's best intentions, her man won't lis-ten or follow through with well-meaning suggestions. If you find your-self in a go-nowhere situation and you feel that you've been spinning your wheels, this chapter will offer hope. You'll read about alternative strategies you can use when your passion-boosting campaigns have hit dead ends.

In Chapter 12, you will learn about situations where your husband's lack of interest in sex with you may not be an indication that he has low sexual desire. He may be involved with masturbation, cybersex and other Internet activities, or infidelity, or he may be confused about his sexual identity. It's important for you to learn about these possibilities so you know where you stand and what you can do to chart your course.

And because no single book can answer all of your questions about boosting and nurturing sexual desire, Part IV provides you with lots of additional helpful resources to help you and your husband achieve the re-sults for which you are hoping. It includes self-help books, methods for finding qualified sex therapists, and useful online resources.

So that's the whole enchilada. Are you up to the task of making real and lasting changes in your sexual relationship? I bet you are! Well, let's get started. Sexier times are right around the corner.

❦ I ❦

All About You

❦

CHAPTER ONE

What Really Goes On Behind Closed Doors:
The *Redbook*-Davis Sexual Desire Poll

Besides helping you create more passion in your marriage, one of the primary reasons I wrote this book is to debunk the hurtful myths about low desire in men. If you believed everything you read or heard about male sexual desire, you would think:

- Most men want sex all the time.
- Low sexual desire is only a woman's problem.
- Some men lack sexual desire, but the prevalence of low desire in men is extremely low.
- Men who aren't interested in sex must have a sexual dysfunction or a serious medical condition. Otherwise they'd be ready to go.

In fact, these are myths, and it can be damaging to believe these are true. As you read these myths, you probably feel exasperated because you know they aren't ture. You also know how damaging it is to believe these untruths. I agree.

When I started writing this book, I tried to do research on the prevalence of low sexual desire in men. What a challenge that was! I discovered that there is precious little research on this topic. When it comes to the subject of low desire in women, that's a different story. Many studies have been conducted on that topic. But even then, the methods used in many of those studies lack scientific rigor and limit confidence in accuracy of the findings. (With all these studies about low desire in women and so few about low desire in men, one has to wonder whether all these researchers are male.)

But perhaps the biggest problem of all is that data about low desire in men are based on self-report. This means that when men are interviewed by perfect strangers, they have to 'fess up and say, "It ain't happening." Do you think that maybe, just maybe, many men might be embarrassed to admit that this is a problem in their lives? Plus, most of these studies don't include collateral reports, meaning feedback from wives. If researchers were to poll women about the quality of their sexual relationship with their husbands, do you think an entirely different picture might be painted?

In terms of the research that is available, here's what we know. The incidence of low libido in men ranges from 0 to 3 percent in some studies to 0 to 15 percent in other studies. Estimates from primary-care and sexuality clinic samples are generally somewhat higher. But when I mulled over these statistics, thought about my own practice, and considered what friends tell me and what their friends tell them, I had nagging doubts about the accuracy of what I was reading. I finally found one relevant study: "Hypoactive Sexual Desire Disorder: An Underestimated Condition in Men" (Eric J. H. Meuleman and J. J. D.M. van Lankveld, *BJU International,* vol. 95, no. 3, Feb. 2005, pp. 291–96). I felt encouraged! These researchers stated, "HSDD [hypoactive sexual desire disorder, or low desire] is more common in men than in women. In public opinion and in medical practice, HSDD is often misinterpreted as ED [erectile dysfunction], and treated as such. There is a need for physicians and patients to be educated, and for the development of reliable clinical tools to assess this aspect of male sexual function." While my own clinical impressions would not lead me to say that there is a higher incidence of low desire in men than women, I found this research compelling.

So I started asking around. I talked to colleagues who are on the front lines working with couples through their marriage and sex therapy practices. They all agreed: low desire appears to be an equal opportunity employer when it comes to gender. If that's the case, then low sexual desire in men has to be America's best-kept secret. (Who knows? It may be the world's best-kept secret!) That's why I decided to team up with *Redbook* and do a survey asking women—not men—about men's sexual desire. *Redbook* loved the idea and we were off and running.

Before we go any further, I want you to know that our survey is not hard scientific research. For one thing, the bulk of the respondents were *Redbook* readers, and we have no idea how representative a *Redbook* reader is in terms of the general population. And although we didn't specify exactly what the poll was about, we did say that it was a sex poll. That could mean that women with sexual issues were drawn to the poll but others were not. However, over 1,000 women responded, and much of what they had to say about their marriages and their sex lives turns conventional wisdom on its head. What they say might not surprise you, but it will certainly help you feel validated.

First, let me tell you a little bit about our questions. We collected demographic information about the women's age, marital status, years married, and number of children. Since this book is about sex-starved wives, we counted only married women's responses.

We asked women questions about their sexual desire, how often they wanted to make love, and the actual frequency with which they made love. We wondered how, from their perspectives, their level of sexual desire compared to that of their husband. We wanted to know who initiated sex more often. We were curious about the percentage of the respondents who described their marriages as sexually compatible versus those who felt out of sync with their partner.

In marriages where mismatched desire was an issue, we questioned how troublesome it was to respondents. Was it "no big deal," slowly degrading their relationships, or somewhere in between? We wanted to know their take on what was causing the sexual chasm: was it sexual dysfunction, personal issues such as depression and fatigue, or relationship issues? We also dared to ask whether they were tempted to go outside their marriages for sexual satisfaction. We were curious about how openly these women discussed their sexual issues with their spouses, friends, and family. We wondered about their willingness to seek help and about the risk of divorce.

Then we asked women to tell us about their husbands. We wanted to know how they thought their men would respond to the same questions asked of them. Although we're well aware that a woman's view of her husband may not accurately reflect how he thinks, feels, and acts, we still believe that her perspective provides valuable information. However, we think our poll holds up an interesting and provocative mirror to married life. Reflecting on the findings, here are some of the highlights. Ready?

- *Sixty precent of the women surveyed said that they were at least as interested in sex as their husbands—and maybe more so.*

Of the 1,004 respondents, 289 women said they were as interested in sex as their husband, and 321 said they were more interested in sex than their husbands. So much for the stereotype that men are always the more interested partner.

- *The "no's" win. Regardless of gender, the person with lower desire regulates the frequency of sex.*

The frequency with which couples actually have sex correlates with the number of times per week the lower-desire spouse desires sex. This reflects with great accuracy what I see in my practice: the person with lower desire has veto power.

- *High-desire wives talk to their husbands about the problem, but their husbands avoid discussing it with them. This is less true of marriages where the roles are reversed.*

Seventy-four percent of high desire women say that they talk to their husbands about their sexual divide, but 55 percent of men never want to discuss it. This must be an incredible source of frustration and resentment on the part of these women.

Imagine what is like to feel devastated by an important part of your relationship and have a partner who does not want to talk about it.

Before you go judging men for being unresponsive, I want to point out once again that shame, frustration, and a sense of failure on the part of men make talking about this sensitive subject very painful.

- *Although 95 percent of high-desire women are either somewhat bothered by the desire gap or consider it to be a serious*

problem in their marriages, 56 percent of them believe that their low-desire husbands aren't bothered by their sexual differences at all.

Women married to low-desire men truly feel that their husbands don't care about sex and aren't troubled by the situation. When one person is upset about something in the marriage and the other person appears unconcerned, it leads to hurt, resentment, and emotional distance.

Couples where the husband has higher desire paint quite a different picture. Women married to high-desire husbands say that 90 percent of their men are either somewhat bothered by the desire gap or consider it to be a serious problem in their marriages, and 78 percent of their wives agree. It helps when both spouses recognize the toll that a sexual divide has on a marriage.

- **About 47 percent of high-desire women ask their husbands to get help, but only 19 percent of their husbands are willing to do so. Twenty-seven percent of high-desire men ask their wives to get help, and 24 percent are willing.**

It's not surprising that women in both kinds of marriages are more willing participants when it comes to seeking help. Nearly all low-desire wives are willing to oblige when their husbands urge them to work on the problem. Fewer than half of low-desire husbands are similarly cooperative. Shame undoubtedly prevents these men from reaching out, but whatever the reason for the resistance to seek help, the marriage unquestionably suffers.

- **High-desire women report feeling at greatest risk of being or having been unfaithful as compared with high-desire husbands, low-desire wives, or low-desire husbands.**

Nearly 37 percent of high-desire women have considered having or have had an affair. Compare this to 24 percent of high-desire men, 19 percent of low-desire women, and 15 percent of low-desire men.

If low-desire men aren't willing to talk about the problem or get help, they leave their wives feeling hopeless, undesirable, and desperate for physical and emotional closeness. Infidelity becomes a very real temptation.

- *Women married to low-desire men initiate sex less frequently than high-desire men do with their wives.*

Although high-desire women crave more sexual contact, when a man is the initiator, he is almost four times more likely to initiate sex than when the high-desire woman is the initiator.

In our culture, men are expected to initiate sex. When they don't, even if women want more sex, they are more reluctant to be the aggressor. And because women stretch outside their comfort zones to initiate sex, they recoil when their initial advances are met with rejection and become gun shy.

High-desire men, in contrast, would much prefer if their wives were more interested. But since men expect to be the initiators, they're more persistent in their attempts to connect.

Although your lower desire girlfriend probably complains that her husband initiates sex regardless of her mood, you have become timid about asserting your needs irrespective of his. You keep telling yourself that he has to be in the mood. After all, his job is a bit more complicated than yours so he needs to be up for it! As you're about to discover, there are many, many ways for you and your husband to experience sexual pleasure together that don't rely on his being in the perfect mood and his penis being up and ready.

- *According to their wives, ED is the cause of low sexual desire in men only 11 percent of the time. The most common causal factors are personal issues, such as depression, fatigue, and stress.*

Most people think that a man's lack of desire is most frequently brought on by an inability to perform. According to the survey, this is not the case. Nonetheless, it's important to point out, that it is also possible that women are not always aware of the extent to which their husbands' anxieties about performance lead to feelings of depression or stress. In other words, women may not always know when ED or premature ejaculation is a precipitating factor of the other personal emotional issues he might be experiencing.

- *In marriages where the man has low desire, nearly 37 percent have sex ranging from once a month to not at all. In marriages*

where women have lower desire, only 20 percent have sex ranging from less than once a month to not at all.

It appears that women married to high-desire men are more sexually active than are low-desire men with their wives.

A few things become clear from these statistics. Women are very interested in sex. (I bet you're relieved to read that!) You're in the majority of women out there who really want a fulfilling physical relationship with their spouses.

If you think that your husband calls the shots when it comes to sexual frequency, he probably does. This is true for most relationships: the person who is less interested sets the pace and tempo of lovemaking.

If you have been troubled by the sexual divide in your marriage and you're having trouble even getting your husband to talk about it, let alone get help for it, it is no surprise to me that you feel like pulling your hair out. According to these findings, one of your husband's least favorite six words probably are, "I want to talk about sex." His least favorite eight words are, "I want you to go to a doctor."

If you have a friend whose sexual desire is lower than yours, you might be surprised how much more receptive she would be to the idea of seeking help. It doesn't necessarily mean that she has a better, more loving marriage; it's just that women are more willing to seek professional help than men are. And generally women are more likely to allow themselves to be influenced by their husbands than the reverse.

So what do you do now? Keep reading, and I'll show you new avenues for enhancing your sexual relationship with the man you love. You deserve a relationship filled with passion, physical intimacy, and emotional connection. I'll help you find your way.

CHAPTER TWO

So, I'm Not Going Crazy After All?

I hope that after reading the previous chapter, you feel better about yourself and your situation. And while knowing that your husband is one of many men for whom sex is not a top priority won't take away your pain, it will help you realize that there's nothing weird, crazy, or abnormal about your reactions. In fact, in this chapter, you will discover how commonplace your feelings really are. See if any of this sounds familiar to you:

> I have started keeping a record in my calendar of when we have sex. In two years, we have had sex on only three dates, and these times have not been very rewarding. There is no intimacy; it always seems to be about him just doing "something" to stop my hurt feelings. He has trouble maintaining an erection, never has an orgasm, and neither do I. Not that an orgasm is the only reason to have sex, but there is no closeness either. It feels as if he is begrudgingly and hastily fulfilling an obligation.

> As a woman who has a husband with a low sex drive, I feel so alone. Often I wonder what is wrong with him. Men aren't supposed to be wired this way. They are the dominant ones, the sex maniacs. So when you have a husband with no drive, you wonder . . . what is wrong. Could he be gay? He is so weird! I feel like

with all the normal men you hear about, how in the world did I find one like this?

Although every woman, man, and relationship is unique, what is not so unique are the thoughts and feelings that stem from a sex-starved marriage. I'm assuming that out of shame or perhaps embarrassment, you probably haven't talked to many people about your husband and your sexual relationship. The first step in improving your sexual relationship is for you to recognize how many other women share your feelings and your concerns. You need to be clear-headed in order to motivate your husband to ramp up his sexual charge; I'm sure you'd agree that you've already had far too many hot-headed arguments about sex. This chapter will help you take the deep breath you've needed for a while.

First, lets talk about self-talk—that little voice inside your head that provides a running commentary on just about everything that's going on in your life. Sometimes you're aware of your inner voice and sometimes you're not, but it's always chattering away. Sometimes the things you say to yourself are positive, and sometimes they're extremely negative. When our inner monologues are negative, we usually end up feeling angry or upset. When they're positive, our outlook tends to be bright. That little voice has a big influence on our mood, how we behave, and how we respond to others.

For example, let's say you make a lovely dinner for your husband, and he's a half-hour late coming home. Do you tell yourself, "Poor guy, he must have gotten caught in traffic. I wish he didn't have such a long drive home every night"? Or do you think, "I can't believe he's late for dinner *again*. He's so inconsiderate. He's undoubtedly out to spite me?" Now imagine how you would feel depending on your inner voice's verdict. What happens the moment your husband walks through the door depends on those feelings.

That little inner voice has lots of power and it affects more than your relationships with other people. You evaluate yourself as well. Most sex-starved wives' self-talk is self-blaming and, more to the point, often off the mark. Just read the following examples of internal dialogue, and you might think I've been camping out in your head.

WHAT WAS I THINKING? I MUST BE STUPID.

Many women have told me that they learned the "love is blind" lesson the hard way. As far back as they can remember, their husbands weren't very sexual. However, these women loved their men, so they wrote off the lack of interest to some external event and forged forward with their relationships. But as time passes, the differences in their interest in sex became glaring:

> I am a thirty-two-year-old woman and will be married for only two (yep, just two) years. Since we have been married, I could probably count the number of times we have had sex on my fingers, and have a few left over. Honestly, by my best estimation, including the honeymoon, the number is something like eight. I am miserable. We dated for about three years prior to getting married. Looking back now, I see that the sex then wasn't all that frequent either, but there always seemed to be reasons, so I did not think there was a problem.

> _____

> My husband was never hot for sex right from the beginning. In fact, I often felt like I was forcing him into it, when it did happen. We've been married for twenty-six years, and until we read *The Sex-Starved Marriage* recently, we hadn't had sex in almost ten years. Gawd, I feel like I am losing it. Any suggestions please?

When this sort of scenario occurs, we tend to look back not only with regret, but with self-condemnation. We tell ourselves that if we were brighter, wiser, more insightful, less dense, we could have spotted the problem long ago and avoided a big mistake. We obsess about "woulda, coulda, shoulda." This self-talk is pointless. It just makes us feel bad about ourselves and drains us of the energy we need to move forward.

It's important for you to recognize that it is extremely common for people to overlook or minimize potential areas of difficulty and emphasize their similarities in the early stages of a romantic relationship. Whether it's the differences in sexual desire, how finances are handled, choices about future children or parenting, decisions about where to live, or how house-

hold chores will be divided, these points of potential conflict get swept under the carpet in favor of focusing on the fun, romance, and excitement that all new relationships bring. There isn't a person alive who can't look back and wonder, "What was I thinking?" regarding some aspect of their marriage in its infancy. In fact, people often tell me that the very thing they loved about their spouse early on is precisely what irritates and annoys them later on in life.

The point is, even if your spouse hasn't changed, your perspective on him often has. You are seeing things differently now, but the operative word here is *now*. Seeing things in a new light requires a new game plan. Stop looking back and berating yourself, and start looking forward to what you can do differently to create more closeness in your marriage.

BUT HE WAS SO SEXY AT FIRST

Some women have the completely opposite experience: they married men who were very sexual in the early part of their marriages. They made love frequently and passionately. But gradually (or not so gradually), things changed; lovemaking became less and less frequent, as did the passion. It wasn't long before these women felt that they were the only ones interested in being close physically.

When we were first married, we both liked sex a lot, and I thought it would always be like that . . . sex in the mornings, before bed, and sometimes when he came from work. Happy, happy me!

It seemed like it didn't take long for him to start to be tired more and more often. I began to notice that it was always me initiating sex, and more and more it seemed like he was just going along with it. It felt like he was performing a household chore, going through the motions, looking for the magic formula too quickly and without much emotional interaction to satisfy me sexually.

Within a couple of years, with each big fight, he would withhold sex for days, weeks, and not talk to me. I would be frustrated and eventually got tired of rejection. I would decide to be nice and friendly but not approach him, and wait . . . and wait and wait (building resentment, hurt, and becoming very cranky). I remember crying quietly to sleep many, many nights.

In between the waves of anger, resentment, and hurt, women come up for air long enough to feel duped. For the life of them, they can't understand why sex used to be so much more important to their husbands. "Is it possible that he just acted as if he were sexual to win me over and convince me to marry him? Is it possible that this was really nothing more than a ploy?"

If you've had these thoughts you've got to know something about human physiology before you jump to conclusions. There may be a biological explanation as to why your sex life has gone downhill. You're undoubtedly aware of the fact that hormones can play a big part in how you feel and on your outlook on life. For example, fluctuating hormones around the time of your period can leave you feeling sad, down, irritable, and angry. You may feel overly sensitive and cry a lot. If this hasn't happened to you, I'm sure you have some friends whose moods feel unpredictable during that certain time of month.

Women aren't the only ones whose hormones fluctuate; men experience their share of hormonal ups and downs too. And if testosterone, one of the primary hormones regulating sex drive, is what's fluctuating, you may be in for a sexual roller-coaster ride. When your spouse has sufficient testosterone in his bloodstream, he is likely to feel vibrant and sexy, have sexual thoughts throughout the day, and find himself fantasizing from time to time. Without sufficient amounts of this hormone, his sexual desire can fade or become nonexistent.

What often happens in the early years of a relationship is that both spouses feel a great sense of infatuation, and infatuation does funny things to hormones. Our brains produce a "love cocktail," and under the influence of these potent brain chemicals, a man with low testosterone experiences a surge in sexual desire. Even if your husband typically has little interest in sex and doesn't get aroused easily, he was ready to go during this heightened period of infatuation. He undoubtedly was thrilled with his new-found sexual energy and told himself, "Now this woman can really turn me on." And you probably thought, "I have finally found someone who enjoys sex as much as I do." (Pat Love, *Hot Monogamy*, pp. 45–46.)

Then, over time, the impact of these hormones faded, and both you and your husband returned to your normal levels of sexual interest, leaving you feeling deceived, and questioning yourself, your husband, or, more commonly, the entire relationship.

It isn't your husband who's played a dirty trick on you; nature has. He is probably as confused as you are about his drop in desire. And although biology might not be the only culprit, a wise woman would not rule it out.

I MUST NOT BE SEXY

As a woman, I felt so damn unpretty. My heart would just physically hurt.

If your husband continually rejects your sexual advances, it won't take long before you start to doubt yourself. Do these questions sound familiar? "Are my boobs too small?" "Have I gained too much weight?" "Am I doing something that turns him off when we do have sex?" "Does he like the way I kiss?" "Has he lost his attraction to me because he doesn't think I'm pretty anymore?" "Have I gotten too old?" "Am I out of shape?" "Does he think other women are sexier than me?" "Does he dislike the way I dress? Is it racy enough for him?" "Does he want me to have plastic surgery?"

Did I forget anything? Has any part of your body escaped your scrutiny? Just fill in the blanks if you've questioned your desirability in ways I haven't already mentioned. And when you're completely done putting yourself down, listen to me.

It is completely understandable that you take your husband's rejections personally. When he says, "Not tonight," you can't help but think that it has something to do with you. And since sexual attraction is often what fuels sexual relationships, how can you think anything other than what you've been thinking? However, here's something you need to know: *your husband's lack of interest in sex may have absolutely nothing to do with you.* I've seen absolutely gorgeous women—10s, for sure—whose husbands routinely avoided sex or even affectionate touching. Any objective observer would agree that these women oozed sexuality. Still, sex wasn't a priority for their mates. To put things in perspective, actress Halle Berry once appeared on

Oprah and discussed her marriage. She was convinced that her husband (who was allegedly a sex addict) turned to other women because she wasn't attractive or sexy enough! Halle Berry!

Another interesting aspect to all of this is that many of the low-libido men I've talked to are completely unaware how their actions hurt their wives. When women initiate sex, the only thing their husbands are thinking about is whether they're in the mood. The husband is not thinking about his wife, her reaction, or the long-term impact on her self-esteem. In fact, many men express surprise when their wives talk about the blow to their hearts or their feelings about themselves. Even when their husbands say repeatedly, "It has nothing to do with you," women don't believe them. And even when women know deep down inside that they're attractive, because other men come on to them, their hurt about their marriages overshadows any positive feelings that might result from other men's interest.

But be aware that your uncertainty about your body or your sexiness might stem from your *own* dissatisfaction with your looks or sexuality. That you're feeling unfit and out of shape maybe is a separate issue from whether your husband has given you specific negative feedback about your body or asked you to change·something for his sake. In Chapter 6, I offer you a plan to tackle these issues and help build your self-confidence.

In the meantime, stop questioning your own desirability. You will soon learn that there are many reasons men lose desire that have absolutely nothing to do with the women in their lives. Once you have more information about this, it will be easier for you to stop blaming yourself and see things more clearly.

I AM UNLOVABLE

I certainly did not feel loved or valued. It often felt that I was stuck with the roommate from hell . . . Now we are separated. And even when things are good between us, he would not/has not initiated lovemaking. If I invite him over and we end up in bed, it is only because I initiate it. I feel like a whore, or something ugly, not loved, not wanted. I feel guilty and ashamed of wanting to have sex.

Perhaps it's not your sexuality you're questioning; maybe you think that you are not lovable as a person. You probably felt completely loved when you met your husband and in the early stage of your marriage. He showered you with attention. You talked for hours and hours. You exchanged loving glances and laughed at the pet names you had for each other. You couldn't wait for the phone to ring when he was away. You felt certain that you had the best friendship ever. You loved him, he loved you, and everything was right in the world.

And in the midst of all this caring, and intimacy, there was touch. You held hands, you caressed each other, and you made love. But then the touching and physical affection stopped. After deciding that you probably weren't sexy enough, you assumed that your husband's withdrawal could not simply be based on his feelings about your sexiness or the shape of your body: you surmised that his rejections were about you as a person. You thought you must not be lovable. Maybe it's your pickiness about how things are done around the house, or the fact that you like to talk more than he does. Maybe it's that you don't make as much money as he does— or maybe you make much more, and he feels emasculated. Maybe he thinks you're angry or depressed, or a nag. Or perhaps you're too outgoing—or not outgoing enough. I'm sure you could come up with quite a list.

Look, the fact that you are longing for touch and physical affection tells me that you are a loving person, that being close is of utmost importance to you. I imagine that there are all sorts of things that are lovable about you as well, and if you think about it for a moment, I know you will agree. In fact, that's what I want you to do right now. Close your eyes, and think about the people in your life with whom you are very close. Now ask yourself, "What do they love about me? What makes me uniquely me that my close friends and family members cherish?" I'm sure you can identify many things about you that are lovable.

However, it's easy to see why constant rejections from your husband leave you feeling that there's something wrong with *you*. But believe it or not, the reasons that your husband may not approach you or be responsive to your advances probably have nothing to do with his feelings of love for you. There's no denying that constant fighting about sex can whittle away intimacy and friendship. But you're about to learn skills that will help you stop fighting and start restoring those loving feelings.

HE'S DOING IT TO GET EVEN

"I saw him as punishing me for something, but who knew what?"

When you're in a relationship and something your partner does hurts you, you are quick to assume that it was done intentionally. This is especially true if you've told your partner about your feelings time and time again but the hurtful behavior persists.

Although it's understandable that your husband's physical and emotional withdrawal can feel punitive, this is not the case in most situations. I know how maddening and frustrating it can feel to have someone be in the position to make unilateral choices that affect you directly. It's so exasperating. And truthfully, it's downright unfair.

Generally the person with the lower sex drive—in this case, your husband—controls the tempo and frequency of the sexual relationship. And to make the situation more challenging, your husband expects you to be okay with his decisions, not to complain, and to continue to be monogamous. But this is an unfair and unworkable arrangement, which is why you feel punished. You have no say in a matter that dearly affects your life.

Nevertheless, it's been my experience that most low-desire men are not out to punish their wives at all. They're more focused on their own emotions, insecurities, or confusion about their lack of interest in sex, and they simply do not fully comprehend the impact on their wives of their actions and the seriousness of the problem.

Sometimes, however, when couples have been fighting about sex for long periods of time, their conflict becomes a secondary problem that takes on a life of its own: the more you want sex, the less he does; the less sexual he becomes, the more determined you are to improve your sexual relationship. You push, he pulls. He pulls, you push.

Once couples get into this tug-of-war dynamic, each spouse resists giving in at all costs, even if giving in means more happiness for both of them. It's human nature to avoid feeling controlled or coerced. Sometimes people cut off their noses to spite their faces to avoid being "told by others what to do."

If this dynamic has occurred in your marriage, you are probably fighting all the time. It may not even be about sex; you find other reasons to argue as well. (Relationships are good for that sort of thing.) Perhaps you have told yourself that the perfect way to make up after one of your arguments is to have sex. Lots of people feel that way. But to your low-desire husband, being physically close when emotions are flaring is probably the last thing he wants to do. For him, it's hard to be close physically when he's feeling distant emotionally.

One disadvantage to believing that your husband is out to punish you is that you will end up feeling angry at him and may treat him in ways that are unkind. Although you might feel some immediate gratification by getting things off your back, spitefulness isn't exactly an aphrodisiac and will push him even further away.

I MUST BE A NYMPHOMANIAC

There must be something wrong with me—I feel like a nymphomaniac. I know I tried talking it out—sharing my feelings, my needs, and always feeling like there was something wrong or freakish about me and my high [sex] drive.

Although there really is such a thing as sexual addiction, most sex-starved wives are not sex addicts; they have completely normal sex drives. Nor do they fit the definition of a nymphomaniac—a woman who, no matter how much sex she gets, can't seem to get enough. No, if you're like most other women in sex-starved marriages, a strong sexual bond is missing, and it's draining the relationship of true intimacy and connection. There's nothing wrong with wanting more of what's good in marriage.

Even so, I can't tell you how many women have told me that they feel that there is something abnormal about them because they want sex more than their husbands do. This feeling is more pronounced when they talk to friends who complain of little or no interest in sex. That's when women with a robust sex drive can really feel odd.

Plus, relationship dynamics are such that the less your husband wants sex, the more you obsess about it. You think about it when you wake up in the morning, when you go to sleep, when you're at work, at the grocery store, when you're reading a book, whenever you're around your husband. Is it any wonder why you question whether you're overly focused on sex? It makes perfect sense to me. Relationships are like seesaws, the more one person does something, the less the other one does of it.

If you're an extremely emotional person, you probably bring out the logical side of your husband. If you're fanatic about tidiness, you're likely to be married to someone who doesn't mind things being disheveled. If you love to socialize whenever possible, your husband is probably more of a loner. It's not that opposites attract (although this is often true), it's just that opposites are created in every relationship over time.

So, although there are probably lots of reasons that your husband has a less-than-robust sex drive that have nothing to do with you or the inter-actions between you, chances are that the tug-of-war—I-need-more-sex versus I'm-not-interested—is sure to play a part in your sexual divide.

Additionally, our culture has an interesting double standard: men with strong sex drives are considered virile, sexy, and manly; women with strong sex drives are often considered "loose" or "slutty." And don't think for a moment that you have escaped this sort of indoctrination. If you've grown up in this kind of culture, you've been socialized to believe in this double standard. However, it's important to remember that you're not wrong, weird, or abnormal because you long for more sex. You understand something very essential about marriage: intimacy is not just icing on the cake; it really is the cake.

I FEEL SO MUCH SHAME

I think we all grow up thinking men always want sex, and it is women who don't. I was too embarrassed to tell people that my own husband couldn't stand to touch me. I felt the need to protect him as well. I would scream horrible things when we fought, but I would never have embarrassed him by even hinting that we had problems.

Most sex-starved wives I see in my practice feel a great deal of shame about their relationships. Because they believe their sex-lite marriage is an exception, they rarely talk to anyone about their hurt and pain. And like the woman above, even though they are aching, many women never reveal to outsiders what really goes on behind closed doors because they are protective of their husbands' egos.

Do you recognize yourself here? If you do, you probably keep your pain, anger, and resentment completely to yourself, where it festers. Futhermore, your shame prevents you from getting the emotional support you sorely need from close friends or family members. It also makes you reluctant to speak to a health care professional, couples therapist, or sex therapist who can help *both* of you find solutions to this dilemma. It's time for you to step out of the closet of shame so that you and your husband reach out and get the help you need.

I FEEL TRAPPED, DEPRESSED, AND ANXIOUS

He always had reasons not to have sex that seemed to be the reasons I *wanted* to have sex: he was stressed, he was tired, he was sick, he was angry. He was always jealous and suspicious that I would find someone else, and to me it seemed he was trying to set that up by withholding so often. I became incredibly depressed and felt trapped with a nearly sexless marriage. I gave myself all kinds of stress-related problems that led to even more distance.

Feeling trapped in a situation can lead to feelings of depression or anxiety because there seems to be no solution. Women in sex-starved marriages feel trapped because they engage in all-or-nothing thinking. They convince themselves that since change in their marriage is impossible, they must either resign themselves to a loveless, sexless marriage or to a divorce, neither of which feels viable. The only other alternative they see is to shut down emotionally—get depressed—or feel incredibly anxious.

Everyone feels depressed or anxious from time to time; that's perfectly normal. But when depression or anxiety becomes chronic, it begins to take an emotional and physical toll. There are many common symptoms of depression and anxiety. You could have trouble sleeping, eating, or concentrating, or you might sleep more or overeat. You might feel unmotivated to do much of anything and find yourself tearful for no apparent reason. As you go through your day, you might notice a feeling of lethargy and overwhelming sadness. If you're more anxious than depressed, you might experience a constant sense of dread and unexplained fear, a feeling of agitation and uneasiness, and find it difficult to focus on day-to-day activities. You could also experience panic attacks.

These are unpleasant feelings and experiences, but relief from these symptoms can be brought about by changing your self-talk. Depressed and anxious people typically engage in extremely negative self-talk: "Things will never change," "I'll never have a good sex life," "Divorce is not an option, but I might as well give up because he'll never understand how I feel about our sexual relationship." These thoughts would make anyone feel depressed!

What typically happens is that instead of focusing on the real issues in the marriage, the depression and the anxiety take main stage. There are trips to psychiatrists, psychotherapists, Barnes & Noble's self-help section, Internet searches for panaceas, depression or anxiety chat rooms, and so on. Until and unless the real issues underlying the feelings of being trapped get resolved, the depression and anxiety will probably linger. Start by using the skills and tools of relationship change you'll find in this book. But if you've been dealing with prolonged sadness, depression, or anxiety, get professional help.

I FEEL SORRY FOR MYSELF AND ANGRY AT HIM

At first I was sympathetic but eventually I became very, very angry and bitter about his robbing me of MY sex life. Neither of us respected the other person's position. He felt pressured, castrated, and belittled by me. I felt punished, hurt, rejected, and I cannot explain the anguish. I know some say, "Don't take it so personally," but it *was* personal. There wasn't anyone else there but me.

When you want something badly and it feels out of your reach because of decisions made by someone else, it's hard not to feel like a victim. This is especially true if you believe you've tried everything, and your husband just doesn't seem to care about your feelings. You think that other women have lively sex lives, and that hurts. You think about your sexual needs not being met and question whether this is how you want to spend the rest of your life.

It's not surprising that you've built up a mountain of self-pity. You tell yourself that you don't deserve this kind of treatment: you're a loving person, and you can't understand why you aren't being treated lovingly in return.

Self-pity and anger are close relatives. If you feel sorry for yourself, you look around for the cause, and he's staring you in the face. (Well, actually, he's probably watching television or reading the newspaper.) And why wouldn't you feel angry? He's depriving you of what you want most: a close, hot, sexual relationship.

But here's the news about self-pity and anger: neither emotion is getting you what you want. Self-pity drains you of energy. I don't just mean energy to try to fix this problem. I mean energy to do anything. It flattens your mood and enthusiasm for life itself.

You don't have to be a rocket scientist to know that anger at your husband won't bring him closer to you; it only pushes him away. Plus, harboring anger and resentment wreaks havoc with your immune system. It can literally make you physically ill. And if you think that unleashing your anger at him is a release, think again. Research tells us that harboring *or* releasing anger just makes you feel angrier.

Whether or not you like it or think it fair, you have to stop having pity parties and hissy fits. You are entitled to feel the way you do—anyone in your shoes would feel that way—but since it's not productive and it will zap you of the get-up-and-go you need to do the work in this book, it's time to take a deep breath and know that once you have a plan, you will feel more empowered and less angry. Here's what one woman said about what happened to her marriage once she gave up feeling sorry for herself:

Ten years ago, I felt like, "poor neglected me. I am unattractive to my husband." Now that attitude is gone because I learned that his low sexual desire is not about me. Accepting his low desire as just a part of the incredible MAN that I married allowed me to ask for what I need without childish pouting and feeling sorry for myself.

This is my response today, after twenty-one years of marriage. I just wish I'd learned these things early on. It could have saved me so many sleepless, lonely nights. It would have saved me the pain of a boob job (thinking THAT would make all the difference . . . duh . . . it's not about me). It would have saved me the fear that I might cheat on him to get my need for feeling loved met. Now I am in control of getting my needs met, and they are getting met! Go figure . . . I guess this is what growing up is all about.

MY MARRIAGE IS HOPELESS

I have expressed my concern for our marriage and our lack of a sex life on many occasions. He admits a problem but does not offer any reason for his disinterest. His patent answer is, "I don't know why." He will not go to counseling. I have brought home many books, which he does not read. He will not speak to a doctor about possible hormonal issues or ED. I have talked 'til I am blue in the face. Nothing. I am at a complete loss.

If I had no sex drive, life would be great. Unfortunately for me, it is not the case. Now I keep my thoughts to myself and show nothing on the outside at all. I am dying inside and don't know how much longer I can hang on.

I know how easy it is to feel hopeless when nothing you've done has helped your situation. I wouldn't be surprised if you've considered separation, divorce, or an affair, or all of these. But when push comes to shove, you know that leaving, either physically or emotionally, isn't exactly what you want. You just want the pain to stop. You want there to be some glimmer of hope that your sexual relationship can be different in the future. You want to believe that someday you will wake up, and all of the distance between you and your husband will have disappeared.

Even though you might be feeling hopeless, here's the truth: if you were entirely hopeless, you wouldn't be reading this book. And you certainly wouldn't have gotten this far. That tells me that even though you've been feeling hurt, misunderstood, and resentful, you're still plugging away. That speaks volumes about you: you're in the ring, fighting for your marriage. To that, I say, "Hats off to you!"

But as you well know, hope isn't enough. You need tools to get through to that man of yours. And since I've helped countless women restore passion, love, connection, and delicious sex in their marriage, I can help you too. Read what a sex-starved woman had to say after reading my last book, *The Sex-Starved Marriage*:

> It's been less than a week since we received the book, and it's already made an incredible difference. We'll be making love tonight for the third time since Friday (and the sex is GREAT!!!). It was exactly the right book at exactly the right time. I think it definitely saved our marriage. Of course, our journey is just beginning, and I'm sure there will be hurdles yet to overcome, but the outlook is now so positive I'm filled with renewed hope.

So allow yourself to feel hopeful. As David Ben-Gurion, a past prime minister of Israel, once said, "Anyone who doesn't believe in miracles isn't a realist."

~II~

Why Men Say No

~

CHAPTER THREE

Physiology Matters

Too many couples are quick to assume that the problems between them are strictly emotional or interpersonal. In other words, if your husband has difficulty maintaining an erection, you might assume it's because he's not attracted to you anymore or that he is angry at you. But his problem may have nothing to do with you; he may in fact find you wildly attractive and have nothing but loving feelings toward you. Physiology might be the only real culprit.

There are many biological reasons your husband may not be interested in sex. These reasons include illness and the the effects of medications that treat it, hormonal problems, and unhealthy lifestyles. Also included in this category are sexual dysfunctions such as erectile dysfunction (ED) and premature ejaculation (PE). Although emotional issues typically arise when a man is struggling with these sexual problems, biology may be a partial or underlying cause. Let's look at some of these issues.

CARDIOVASCULAR DISEASE

Cardiovascular disease kills sexual desire. It blocks arteries, and when blood flow is insufficient, men have difficulty getting and maintaining erections. In addition, without proper blood flow, a man's penis will not be as sensitive to touch. All of this leads to frustration and feelings of inadequacy in the bedroom, which undoubtedly affects sexual desire.

ENDOCRINE DISORDER

Endocrine disorders such as diabetes, hypothyroidism, and hyperprolactinemia can affect sexual desire. Hyperprolactinemia is an uncommon disorder in which too much of the hormone prolactin is produced by the pituitary gland. Ten percent of men experiencing low sexual desire have prolactin-secreting pituitary tumors. A loss of interest in sex may be the first sign of a pituitary problem.

Diabetes often results in reduced testosterone levels in men, and testosterone is one the primary hormones responsible for sex drive. Additionally, there is often an increased sense of pain during sex associated with neuropathy, a condition of the nervous system common in diabetes. Decreased sexual desire can occur from the medications taken for high blood pressure, depression, pain, and weight control often associated with diabetes.

An improperly functioning thyroid frequently causes sexual problems. The thyroid gland can be underactive (hypothyroidism) or overactive (hyperthyroidism). It is estimated that over two-thirds of the men with hypothyroidism experience low sexual desire, premature ejaculation, and delayed ejaculation. Among the men with hyperthyroidism, 50 percent experience premature ejaculation, 17 percent report having low sexual desire, and 15 percent experience ED.

CHRONIC ILLNESS

Any chronic illness can take its toll on sexual desire: liver disease, kidney disease, pituitary disease, Parkinson's disease, anemia, and arthritis, among others. Chronic pain can take a toll too.

ALCOHOLISM AND ABUSE OF DRUGS

Many times people think that alcohol enhances one's sex life because it reduces inhibitions. Although a small amount of alcohol might be relaxing, drinking excessively creates sexual problems. Your husband might have difficulty getting and maintaining erections and difficulty ejaculating, all of which could dampen his desire.

Additionally, excessive alcohol consumption (more than two beers a day, two glasses of wine, or one mixed drink) can significantly increase prolactin, which leads to prostate and breast enlargement in men, as well as resulting in lower sexual desire. Drinking wine in moderation or becoming abstinent can help restore sexual desire. For problem drinkers, alcoholism, and other addictions (marijuana, cocaine, heroin, painkillers), professional help should be sought.

Smoking is bad for sexual health as well. Tobacco impairs circulation and makes achieving an erection more difficult.

MEDICATIONS AND MEDICAL TREATMENTS

Medications can greatly affect sex drive. Antidepressants, antihistamines, tranquilizers, and antihypertensive, antipsychotic, antiarrhythmic, and anticonvulsant medications can all lower desire. The side effects of chemotherapy can have an impact on libido too, as well as medicines used for prostate problems.

TESTOSTERONE FLUCTUATIONS

When a man experiences a drop in sexual desire, insufficient levels of testosterone may be part of the problem. The U.S. Food and Drug Administration (FDA) estimates that 4 to 5 million American men may suffer from low testosterone, but only 5 percent are treated. Again, low testosterone levels can cause low sexual desire, ED, reduced muscle mass and strength, osteoporosis, depression, and fatigue.

MALE MENOPAUSE

As women, we're constantly saturated with facts and figures about peri-menopause, menopause, and the various hormonal changes that accompany them and how they affect our sex drive. But we really don't hear about men and the hormonal changes men experience. Have you ever heard of "andropause," or androgen deficiency of the aging male (ADAM), also known as male menopause? Andropause refers to hormonal and physiological changes in men ages forty to fifty-five, though some experts say it can occur as early as thirty-five or as late as sixty-five. A drop in testosterone and other hormones characterizes this stage. These hormonal changes often lead to depression, weight gain, *and* a decreased sex drive, which is the most common symptom. And you probably don't know this, but andropausal men can also experience hot flashes, sweats, nervousness, and fatigue.

OBESITY

In one study, obese people were twenty-five times as likely to report dissatisfaction with their sex lives as normal-weight people. They cited problems in at least one of four areas: lack of sexual enjoyment, lack of sexual desire, difficulty with performance, and avoidance of sexual encounters.

SLEEP PROBLEMS

Shakespeare once said that sleep is "the balm of hurt minds, great nature's second course, chief nourisher in life's feast." Unfortunately, not everyone is fueled by this sort of nature's nourishment. It's estimated that about one-third of all Americans don't sleep very well. We all have a night or two when we are tossing and turning and can't quite shut off our brains; this is nothing to be alarmed about. However, long-term sleep deprivation can lead to feelings of anxiety, nervousness, depression, lowered resistance, and a reduced sex drive.

LACK OF EXERCISE

Does your husband work out regularly? If he expects to feel sexy, he should. Even a brief aerobic workout can help him feel more desire and strengthen his orgasms. That's because exercise increases endorphins, or "feel good" chemicals, which last for about an hour after a short workout session. In one study, seventy-eight sedentary men were asked to exercise for sixty minutes a day, three days a week, for nine months. Participants in the study felt sexier, initiated sex more, and enjoyed it more.

SEXUAL DYSFUNCTION

One of the primary reasons men avoid sex is that they're experiencing sexual problems such as erectile dysfunction and ejaculation problems. According to a large study published in the *Journal of the American Medical Association*, about a third of men said they had persistent problems with sex. ("Sexual Dysfunction in the United States," Edward O. Laumann, Anthony Paik, Raymond C. Rosen, 1999.) Although I have included information about sexual dysfunctions in this chapter, when it comes to erectile dysfunction and problems with ejaculation, there is a complex interplay among biological, emotional, and interpersonal causal factors.

Erectile Dysfunction
Erectile dysfunction (ED) is the inability to achieve or maintain an erection long enough to have mutually satisfying intercourse. Difficulty getting or maintaining erections is very common; most men experience it at some point in their lives. It is not a cause for concern, however, unless it is persistent. It's also common for men to experience changes in their erections as they get older; they typically take more time and more stimulation to achieve an erection, their orgasms are often less intense, there is less ejaculate, and they need more time before they're able to achieve another erection. All of this is normal.

It is estimated that approximately 30 million American men deal with ED. Some men have struggled with this issue throughout their lives. Others have had perfectly normal sex lives in the past, only to encounter ED later in life. The study by Laumann, Paik, and Rose showed that men aged fifty to fifty-nine are three times more likely to experience ED than men aged eighteen to twenty-nine.

Biology is not the only reason men experience ED; stress, anxiety, guilt, depression, low self-esteem, unhappy childhood experiences, and unresolved relationship issues can wreak havoc with a man's ability to achieve erections. Furthermore, regardless of the primary cause of ED, once a man has difficulty getting or maintaining an erection, it will undoubtedly affect how he feels about himself, his sexuality, and his ability to make love. He may begin to experience anxiety about failure, which can (and often does) worsen ED.

Underlying conditions such as kidney disease, chronic alcoholism, multiple sclerosis, atherosclerosis, diabetes, and cardiovascular disease cause men to have difficulties getting or maintaining erections. Injuries to the penis, pelvis, spinal cord, prostate, and bladder can be contributing factors. Surgery for cancer of the prostate is another culprit. Side effects from many medications including high blood pressure drugs, antihistamines, and antidepressants, can disrupt blood flow in the genitals, which often causes ED.

There are several tests a doctor can perform to identify whether an underlying physical condition is causing ED. A doctor can also help determine if nonphysical issues are the primary causes. Since most men naturally get erections in their sleep, a simple test can confirm whether this is occurring. If a man is in fact having nocturnal erections, the problem is more likely to be a psychological one.

At the risk of repeating myself, if your husband is having problems getting or maintaining erections, I know you'll be doubting your attractiveness, lovability, and even your value as a person. And when you're not putting yourself down, you'll be driving yourself crazy with other explanations for his inability to make love to you. Remember: his sexual dysfunction may have *absolutely nothing to do with you*. Your husband may be wrapped up in his own thoughts, insecurities, and fears, and his withdrawal from you may be the only way he can protect himself from an overwhelming sense of failure. You'll find a section in Chapter 7 that deals with ways to cope with ED.

Premature Ejaculation

An even more common sexual problem is premature ejaculation (PE). In fact, it is *the* most common sexual dysfunction for men. Premature ejaculation means that men ejaculate earlier than they (or their partners) would like—before, upon, or shortly after penetration. Some men struggle with PE throughout their sexually active lives, while others develop problems in later life. Keep in mind that what is considered premature is very subjective. If a man ejaculates after ten minutes of intercourse and his wife has had an orgasm after nine minutes, all is right in the world. If our ten-minute-man is married to a woman who takes fifteen minutes to orgasm, they both may feel dissatisfied with his staying power. And if a woman takes an exceptionally long time to be satisfied, a man's ejaculating before she reaches orgasm might not be considered PE at all: rather, it may be more an issue of delayed orgasm for the woman.

Often, when a man ejaculates quickly, he typically feels shame and anxiety about his ability to perform. PE can also cause relationship problems because satisfying intercourse is not likely. Studies suggest that at least 30 percent of men grapple with this problem on a regular basis. However, various surveys suggest that the incidence of PE is probably considerably higher because men don't like to admit having this difficulty.

Not surprisingly, when a man persistently ejaculates before he would like, he is going to be uptight when he is making love; he will probably have a hard time becoming aroused and will be less likely to enjoy himself. And it makes sense that if sex isn't enjoyable, he is going to want to steer clear of it.

DEALING WITH PHYSICAL CAUSES

If you suspect that biology may play a part in your husband's lack of interest in sex, he should start with a visit to a physician who can rule out physical causes. Sometimes there are simple solutions—a change in medication, a lifestyle change, diagnosing and treating an underlying medical condition—that can quickly improve his libido and get your love life back on track.

If you're thinking, "I've tried that already. He won't go," or, "He's been to his doctor; he just won't follow through with the doctor's suggestions," Relax. I'm going to help you get through to him. On my Web site sexstarvedwife.com, I've created a special section for men only. There he'll find the things he needs to know about you, your need to have a more sexually satisfying relationship, and what he has to do to step up to the plate and take responsibility for making things better between you. This will include, among many other things, a strong nudge to go see a doctor.

You might think that you've said the same things to him before without positive results, and it's possible that your husband might respond to my words in the same way. However, it's been my experience in my extensive work with couples, and in my own marriage for that matter, that sometimes other people's words carry more weight. You probably know what I mean. How many times has it happened that you've made a suggestion to your husband that goes in one ear and out the other, but when a friend or relative says exactly the same thing, your husband thinks the idea is brilliant? Infuriating, isn't it? Plus, your stubborn husband just might feel that there's something significantly different about taking advice from an author than from his wife with whom he's been at odds over this subject. So let me talk turkey to your husband, and I will try to chip away at his defensiveness and uncover the caring I know he has about you and your marriage.

In addition to biological factors, your husband might be coping with some troubling personal issues that have driven his libido underground. The next chapter takes a look at some of these libido-lowering issues.

CHAPTER FOUR

It's All About Him

You just read about the physiological causes of low desire; in this chapter, we'll explore the personal issues that your husband might be coping with. Here are the most typical libido busters.

BODY IMAGE

My wife was afraid of the dark . . . then she saw me naked and now she's afraid of the light.

—Rodney Dangerfield

Do you think women are the only ones who are obsessed with having perfect bodies or get depressed when they look in the mirror and don't exactly love what they see? Wrong! Although men are usually a little easier on themselves than we are, don't kid yourself; men won't win the Good Housekeeping Seal of Approval for Self-Acceptance. No, men struggle with their self-images too. They want to look great physically, and they're paying big bucks to make it happen. Like us, men get nose jobs, breast reductions, pectoral implants, hair implants, eyelid surgery, facelifts, botox injections, and liposuction.

My husband subscribes to the popular and well-respected magazine *Men's Health.* Have you ever seen the cover of that magazine? It's always the same: an incredibly buff, handsome man with six-pack abs graces each month's cover. I don't think it's the same guy every month, but who can tell? Who looks at his face? And that's precisely the point. This body-building cover boy lures men to buy the magazine with the hope that they can become body beautiful too.

Women don't have a corner on the "I hate my body" market; men are vain too, although they might not talk about it as much as we do. Your husband may feel bad about the ten pounds he's put on this year, but he's unlikely to ask, "Do I look fat in these jeans?" It's important for you to keep in mind that simply because your husband doesn't express his unhappiness with his body doesn't mean that he isn't unhappy. And if he thinks he's fat, ugly, skinny, or not buff enough, he's probably not feeling all that sexy. When a person doesn't feel good about his body, who wants to be touched? Each touch triggers self-consciousness and a feeling of discomfort rather than feelings of pleasure and delight. Shame or self-disgust block feelings of sensuality or desire.

Is it possible that your husband is feeling bad about his body and that these feelings have gotten in the way of his feeling sexual? If you're not sure, here are some questions to ask yourself:

- Has he made negative statements about his body?
- Has he allowed himself to indulge in unhealthful foods that have added pounds to his middle?
- Are there parts of his body that he doesn't like?
- Has he accepted the changes in his body that aging often brings, or has that gotten him down in the dumps?
- Have long hours at the gym and ever-growing muscles made you wonder if he will ever be satisfied with his body, or is a good body image just a moving target?
- Is he taking steroids or other drugs to build muscle or reduce fat?
- Has he developed strange eating habits that have made you wonder whether he's anorexic or bulimic?

If you answered yes to any of these questions, your husband may be feeling crappy about his body. In addition to not feeling sexy, research tells us that when people dislike their bodies, they generally have low self-esteem. It's hard to know which comes first, the chicken or the egg, but for our purposes, it really doesn't matter. What matters is that you understand that if he's feeling bad about himself, he won't have much energy for sex. What can you do to help him with this? Plenty. The solutions are in the Chapters in Part III. You're almost there.

NOT FEELING MANLY

Do you remember the book, *Real Men Don't Eat Quiche*? Tongue-in-cheek, this little book defined what it meant to be a 1980s man in our culture. Follow the rules, and you're masculine. Disregard the rules, and you're a sissy. Although the rules have changed a bit, there are still hard-and-fast definitions for what it takes to be a man. And it's not just well-defined abs.

In our culture, a real man must be tough, strong—both emotionally and physically—independent, aggressive, decisive, in charge, financially successful, and tight-lipped about his innermost feelings. Additionally, he must have a high sex drive, impressive sexual prowess, and a penis that, like the Energizer bunny, just won't quit. If he falls short of any of these expectations, he feels less of a man.

Whether or not you buy into these limiting and unreasonable stereotypes is not the point. If your husband measures himself by them and doesn't feel he quite measures up, he might not feel manly enough to be in the mood for sex. He (and you) will need to reexamine these self-limiting beliefs in order for him to feel more masculine—and therefore sexier.

STRESS

When we detect an emergency—an attack, threat, or harm—our bodies protect us by producing chemicals that enable us to run or fight. Unfortunately, our bodies respond the same way to a dangerous situation in a dark alley and spending too many hours on the job: we feel tense, vigilant, and anxious.

Stress takes a toll on us both emotionally and physically. We feel burned out, fatigued, irritable, and uptight. And if we feel this way long enough, we become sick, depressed, and even accident prone. Stress zaps the joy out of life because we're always in a knot. For many people, stress triggers a definite drop in sexual desire.

How can you tell if your husband is stressed out? Does he work long hours and seem preoccupied when he comes home? Does he feel overburdened by responsibilities, real or imagined? Does he frequently seem edgy around the kids? Does he have a short fuse when you're around him? Is he drinking or smoking more to try to calm his nerves? Has he been engaging in self-destructive behavior that endangers his health? Is he worrying about finances, family members, or world affairs?

If your answer to any of these questions is yes, your husband's stress levels may have gotten the best of him. He might not discuss his feelings of stress with you—many men keep their problems to themselves—but he may be affected by them nonetheless. In fact, if he has no outlets for relieving stress such as exercise, and believes that he must deal with his feelings alone, stress can accumulate.

You might say to yourself, "If he feels stressed out, why not just jump in bed? That would be a great way to relax." Although there are many people who would agree with you, it just so happens that your husband isn't one of them. Some people love sex when they're tense because it relaxes them; others must be relaxed in order to enjoy sex.

JOB LOSS

Has your husband lost his job and seemed down for far longer than you might have expected? Have you had a hard time understanding why he isn't picking himself up by his bootstraps and moving on with his life despite his disappointment? Has his joblessness triggered a host of other problems, including health difficulties or depression? Does he seem cynical or hopeless about the future? Has his self-esteem plummeted out of sight? Has he been edgier than normal around you? Many men struggle emotionally when they become unemployed.

You might not understand why your man is having trouble bouncing back from his job loss. After all, you've experienced losses in your life, and they may not have hit you so hard. But I want you to know that in my years working with couples, involuntary unemployment, especially for older men, can be nothing short of devastating. And unfortunately, it's been my experience that many women can't really appreciate their husbands' pain. If this is true for you, let me help you gain some perspective.

In our culture, although two-career families are becoming the norm, we still expect men to be the primary breadwinners. Most men's self-esteem is inextricably connected to their employment success. Most women, on the other hand, evaluate themselves on the basis of their success with relationships; this is true even of women who have top-level, high-powered careers. So when a man is released from his position at work, it's not simply a job that he is losing; it's his sense of self, and that's a mighty hard hit. Many women can better understand this feeling by comparing it to how they feel when relationships fail. Naturally this description of gender roles is quite stereotypical and may not apply to your marriage. However, if your husband has shut down emotionally after a loss of a job, it's because his sense of identity and masculinity has really been called into question; he feels insecure and uncertain about his future. Sex is not a top priority. In fact, it may not even be on his list of priorities at all. This will change, but it will require patience and understanding on your part.

DEPRESSION

Everyone gets depressed once in a while. Something happens that we don't like, and we feel down in the dumps. A little while later—after a few hours, days, or weeks—we're up and running again. This sort of depression is unlikely to interfere in any significant way with your day-to-day existence or your marriage. But that's not the kind of depression I'm talking about here. I'm talking about clinical depression, a debilitating condition that affects approximately 18 million American adults, or 10 percent of the population, in any given year.

There are several kinds of depression. Dysthymia is a chronic low-grade depression. People who suffer from dysthymia go about their lives feeling blue, hopeless, and unhappy. They have a hard time concentrating and often feel low self-esteem. Unfortunately, because the symptoms are uncomfortable but not debilitating, many of these people do not get the help they need, and the feelings of depression can last for years, even decades. But make no mistake about it: just because the symptoms of depression are considered mild, long-standing depression takes its toll, affecting sleep, eating habits, and energy. It can lead to a more severe depression or even suicide. To warrant the diagnosis of dysthymia, your husband must have been feeling depressed for at least two years.

With major depression the most severe kind of depression, the symptoms are more intense and usually interfere with a person's life. A major depression can be the result of a traumatic event, or the accumulation of many of life's disappointments or bad experiences. Sometimes people don't know why they feel depressed; they just do. When people are in the throes of major depression, it is fairly obvious because the quality of life for that person and that person's loved ones undergoes a radical shift.

If you're wondering whether your husband may be depressed, here are some signs to look for:

- Feelings of sadness, anxiety, remorse, pessimism, worthlessness, or emptiness, lasting for at least two weeks
- Inability to make decisions or feeling helpless to change anything
- Changes in sleeping habits (sleeping many more hours or insomnia)
- Chronic fatigue and lack of motivation
- Changes in eating habits (overeating or loss of appetite)
- Weight loss or gain
- Crying
- Inability to concentrate
- Irritability
- Frequent thoughts of suicide

If you think your husband is depressed, I know it has been hard on you, especially if you've never experienced depression yourself. You have a hard time believing that he really wants to feel better and can't fathom why he seems so unmotivated to take the necessary steps to feel better. You wonder if he is punishing you with his emotional absence. You feel lonely and helpless as you watch your husband let his life slip through the cracks.

There's no question that living with a depressed spouse is difficult. Being clinically depressed is like being in a black hole with no sign of light anywhere; things that once gave pleasure lose all meaning, and the future seems to be nothing more than a miserable extension of these dark days. People who are depressed also have a hard time recalling better times in the past. They feel dead inside, and sometimes just making it through the day is a major feat; indeed, many report having difficulty getting out of bed in the morning. Simple day-to-day tasks like taking a shower or shaving become major chores. Despite what it might seem on the outside, people don't choose to be depressed. It's lonely and frightening. Freeing oneself from depression is hard work.

Seventy-five percent of people who are depressed confirm a loss of sexual desire. And to add insult to injury, as I mentioned earlier, antidepressants are well known for their effects with arousal, orgasm, ejaculation, or erectile difficulties.

There are other forms of depression as well. To read more on this topic, I highly recommend Michael Yapko's books, *Breaking the Pattern of Depression* or *Hand Me Down Blues.*

GRIEF

If we live long enough, we will experience loss. Whether it's the death of a loved one, the loss of a significant relationship, a pet, a job, physical capabilities, or children leaving home, loss is inevitable. Grief is a normal response to loss. The larger the loss, the greater the grief can be.

Someone who is grieving is often consumed with sadness. Little else matters. Thoughts about the impact of the loss or past memories are played over and over in the mind of the grieving person. Concentration on daily matters becomes challenging. Those who grieve also often feel guilt, remorse, and anxiety. They frequently avoid socializing or interacting with others. Many seem angry or irritable. As with depression, grief can result in physical symptoms such as fatigue, changes in sleeping and eating patterns, or a total loss of interest in sex.

If your husband has experienced a loss recently, chances are his lack of desire is brought about by his suffering. Grief has no universal timetable;

everyone grieves differently and for different lengths of time. Even though you think he should be over his sadness, it has to run its course. Sometimes professional help is needed to assist him through his pain. Have him read the chapter I've devoted to men on sexstarvedwife.com.

MIDLIFE CRISIS

Let me set the record straight: men today aren't waiting until midlife to have their midlife crises; they're often doing it in their thirties and forties. I tell you this because I'm afraid that if your husband is younger, you'll be tempted to skip over this section. Don't. Your younger man might just fit the midlife crisis bill.

Were you thinking that your marriage is sound despite the usual ups and downs and then all of a sudden your husband tells you that he is unhappy? But he means that he's *really* unhappy, as in, "I love you, but I'm not in love with you anymore." And when you ask for clarification, that's when he tells you that he's never been happy in the marriage. You're too fat, too thin, too critical, too demanding, too this or too that. The worst part is that he's convinced that the key to his unhappiness is getting out of the marriage. But he doesn't run out and contact a lawyer just yet. He simply growls in the corner; busies himself with work, hobbies, his computer, or _____ (fill in the blank); pulls himself away emotionally; and avoids you like the plague. Sex is absolutely out of the question.

Sometimes it's easy to spot a man who's in a midlife crisis. He's the guy who does it the conventional way. He notices his bulging stomach, his graying hair (if he still has any), and his fading eyesight and realizes that he is no longer the youthful warrior he once imagined himself to be. So he buys a red convertible sports car, has an emotional or physical affair with a younger woman, joins a gym and works out like a fanatic, listens to his teenage son's CDs, buys a flashier wardrobe, and, in the hopes of proving to himself that he is in fact immortal, takes up a new death-defying hobby like hang gliding.

Then there are the guys who enter this phase with more reserve, self-doubt, and introspection. They may look at their lives and accomplishments and wonder, "Is this all there is?" They may wake up one morning to the epiphany that they've been following the rules for so long that they wonder what life would be like if they just followed their bliss and grabbed for the gusto. They ponder the True Meaning in Life. And in the midst of all this existential angst, one thing is for sure—sex just isn't happening.

CULTURAL AND RELIGIOUS INFLUENCES

Healthy sex is a natural, wonderful, and pleasurable experience. When spouses enjoy their sexual relationship, they say that sex is the tie that binds. But for some people, sex is rarely, if ever, enjoyable. Instead of focusing on the physical pleasure or emotional intimacy that sex can bring, these folks experience guilt, shame, anxiety, or physical discomfort, along with an inability to relax and have an orgasm. Those who have unpleasant feelings before, during, or after a sexual encounter are unlikely to want to do that again.

Why do some people recoil at the thought of sex? The answer is complicated. But one common reason people are uncomfortable with sex is their upbringing. It's possible that your husband grew up in a family in which sex was portrayed as being bad or "dirty." If he learned from his parents or his religious upbringing that sex is sinful, he might have been shamed or punished for having sexual feelings or for masturbating. Even if his parents never said a word about sex, imagine the lessons your husband learned as a little boy if they never showed any outward signs of affection in his presence. You husband may be struggling with these issues silently.

SEXUAL, EMOTIONAL, OR PHYSICAL ABUSE

If your husband had the great misfortune to grow up in a home where family members were physically or emotionally abusive, it might have corroded his sense of trust, security, and comfort in the world. He might have created emotional defenses to protect himself from hurt. It's hard to be intimate when you have an impenetiable wall wrapped around you.

This sort of armor precludes having a warm, loving, sensual, sexual relationship.

And what if the unspeakable happened and your husband experienced sexual abuse as a child or a young man? How does this affect his psyche and his sense of himself as a sexual being? Millions of men have experienced abuse at the hands of an older person—an immediate or extended family member, neighbor, stranger, a trusted teacher or religious leader. Often the perpetrator was a man, but not always. Sometimes the abuse was a single event, and sometimes it was ongoing. Often the victim is told that if he talks to someone about the abuse, he will be punished. This admonition, along with shame, prevents many young boys from disclosing the truth about their experiences. In fact, victims of abuse often feel so much shame that they never reveal their past to anyone. But secrecy doesn't protect; it often exacerbates the shame. Although not everyone who has experienced sexual abuse will struggle with sexual issues, it is nonetheless a common outcome. This is especially true for those who have not adequately dealt with the possible emotional fallout from such an experience.

In addition to sexual abuse, many young boys experiment sexually when they're young, and, frequently, this is same-sex experimentation. This sort of experience does not necessarily mean that the boy is gay or that he will be in the future. But often there is confusion and guilt about these sexual incidents, and these negative feelings can be carried into adulthood.

Emotional abuse as a child can also wreak havoc on a man's sexuality. If family life was erratic, hurtful, or scary, he probably learned at a young age that it's not safe to feel close. Instead, he learned that relationships are unpredictable at best. And since genuine physical closeness involves vulnerability, it may be far too threatening to someone who learned that vulnerability leads to harm.

If your husband has had any of these life experiences, they may still have a stubborn stronghold on him unless he has found healthy ways of integrating them into his life. He will need to learn how to shake free from the past so that he can be emotionally, physically, and spiritually present with you.

SEXUAL ORIENTATION CONFLICT
OR CONFUSION

Marie was at a loss. She and her husband, David, had been married for seventeen years and had two children. Although Marie had always been more sexual than David, she accepted their differences and felt good about their marriage nonetheless. However, during the past few years, David's interest in sex had waned; they had stopped making love completely. Marie probed and probed, but David revealed nothing.

One day while Marie was straightening up their bedroom, she came across a magazine for gay men. She was shocked. After several hours of catching her breath, she called David at work and asked him to come home to talk with her about something important. Since David owned his own business, he had flexibility and returned home quickly. Marie confronted him with the magazine and asked why he had it. David made no attempt to create excuses or to lie to Marie. He told her that he had been confused about his sexual identity for many years. He found himself attracted to men, but because he loved her and loved his children, he couldn't bring himself to tell her about this because he didn't want his family life to end. He had decided to stop having sex with Marie when he could no longer stand the conflict. Although Marie was devastated, she was relieved to get the truth and to begin to understand what was really going on in her marriage and why their sexual relationship had ended.

Based on a study from the New York City Health Department, it is estimated that 10 percent of men who identify themselves as straight have sex only with other men. And 70 percent of those straight-identified men having sex with men are married. In fact, 10 percent of all married men in this survey reported same-sex behavior during the past year.

If you have wondered whether your husband might be gay or bisexual, you wouldn't be alone. For many reasons, not the least of which is health issues such as contracting sexually transmitted diseases, if you are truly concerned, it's essential that you address this issue openly and honestly. I realize that may be hard to do, but if your husband is living a lie, it's not good for him, you, or anyone else in your family.

SEXUAL COMPULSIONS

Is your husband staying up late at night and visiting pornographic Web sites? Does he peruse pornographic magazines regularly but refuse to come to bed with you? Although he tells you that he's lost interest in sex or that he's just too tired to respond to your sexual advances, do you repeatedly find telltale signs that he's been masturbating? If so, your husband may be engaging in sexually compulsive behaviors.

There are many people who look at pornographic magazines, read sexually titillating books, or view X-rated videos, and these behaviors don't in any way interfere with their sexual relationship or their lives. In fact, for some, moderate use of these materials can enhance sexuality. But there are those who abuse or overuse these sexually charged materials, and the behavior can become a compulsion.

People who act compulsively often want to stop or limit their time engaged in sexual behaviors but feel they cannot. In fact, they may end up spending increasing amounts of time participating in the sexually charged activities. More of their conscious awareness during the course of the day goes into planning, executing, and recovering from sexual behavior. Frequently those with sexual compulsions continue engaging in the sexual activity despite the fact that they are causing personal, relational, or career problems. In other words, despite their best intentions, their compulsion takes priority. As a result, people may become neglectful of personal and professional responsibilities. Additionally, they may spend large amounts of money to support the habit. They may frequent strip clubs, purchase expensive subscriptions to pornographic Web sites, or even pay for sex.

Some people develop compulsive sexual behavior to quell underlying feelings of stress, anxiety, boredom, unhappiness, or loneliness. And because engaging in sexual behavior actually changes one's biochemistry—"feel good" chemicals and hormones are released—many professionals believe that becoming sexually aroused and having an orgasm can be seen as a form of self-medication. But this sort of "therapy" stands in the way of people developing healthier solutions to life's disappointments. And the more time a man spends with a computer, magazines, or videos, the less time and energy he has left for his wife or other meaningful activities or people.

If your husband is avoiding sex with you but has an active sexual life on his own, you're entitled to feel neglected. This isn't the way healthy sexual relationships are meant to be. However, feeling like a victim won't get you very far. In Chapter 6, I'll help you better understand what you're dealing with and, more important, how to influence your husband to change.

SEXUAL OR EMOTIONAL INFIDELITY

Unfortunately, many women correctly suspect that the primary reason their husbands aren't interested in sex is that they're having an affair. The affair may be strictly emotional—they may see each other at work, have meals together, share intimate secrets, secretly spend time together—or it may include being sexual—heavy petting, oral sex, or intercourse. Either way, there is a betrayal.

An illicit relationship demands time and energy for planning, covering up, fantasizing, meeting, and covering up some more. Then throw in time for guilt, remorse, justification, shame, excitement, and what's left for a marriage? Zilch. Frequently people in the throes of affairs feel so guilty or are so busy justifying their behavior to themselves that they simply cannot face their spouse, let alone make love to them. And of course they may be getting their emotional or sexual needs met outside the marriage.

Do any of these personal issues ring a bell with you? If so, pay particular attention to the solutions devoted to resolving personal issues in Chapter 6. You will find some suggestions as to what you can do differently to help your spouse begin to deal with some of his personal demons.

But if you don't think that your husband's personal issues are what's keeping you apart, his lack of interest in sex may have something to do with relationship issues, the subject of the next chapter.

CHAPTER FIVE

A Couple's Conundrum

If, after reading the previous two chapters, you aren't completely clear on the reasons your husband has retreated sexually, perhaps this chapter will provide the missing link. This chapter offers you a look into some of the relationship factors that often play a part in sexual meltdowns. Even if biological or personal issues are the primary causes of his lack of desire, when a desire gap has been long standing, there will undoubtedly be relationship fallout. Read this chapter carefully, because it will help you determine which areas of your marriage need your attention. Then Chapter 11 will help you decide what to do about these issues.

Don't kiss me like we're married, kiss me like we're lovers.
—K. T. Oslin

I wish I had a dollar for each time a woman has told me that her sexual relationship went down the tubes as soon as she and her husband got married. Prenuptially, they really had it going on. Everything was intense—their kisses, loving glances, flirtatious banterings, lingering touches—everything. But once they tied the knot, everything changed.

If this has happened in your marriage, you could be married to a man whose feelings of sexuality are triggered by mystery, adventure, and romanticism. Although familiarity offers great comfort to most people, it might be a major desire buster for your husband. The more comfortable he's grown with you because of your committed relationship, the less aroused he feels. You can be his wife or his sex kitten, but not both. "Wife" becomes synonymous with sedate, safe, and stifling, not the stuff his fantasies are made of.

THE NOT-SO-HOT MAMA

What's a not-so-hot mama? If a woman's becoming a wife changes things for a man, having children can have an even bigger impact. Was sex fairly hot between the two of you before your kids came, but all that changed drastically once you got pregnant or when your children were born? You're not alone. In the same way that some men have a hard time feeling sexual about their wives, others can't reconcile having hot sex with a pregnant woman or a mom, even if she happens to be the mother (or mother-to-be) of his children. In their minds, motherhood and eroticism just don't quite jibe.

> I would say that my husband (nearly fifteen years of marriage) has very little interest in touch right now. That includes sex. We have not made love for nearly a year. What has changed?
>
> Our daughter was born last February. When my husband saw the twenty-week ultrasound, that was the start of the end to our sex life. He said, "Our little daughter is in there." But after the birth, we made love once or twice, a couple of months after she was born, and that was it!

If your husband is the queasy sort who saw you giving birth, he might not be able to get some of those images out of his mind. Your vagina, whose sole job it once was to welcome his sexy penis, has now been transformed into a birth canal. Then to top it off, your beautiful, sensual breasts that he has always loved to touch, kiss, and suck—once the titillating objects of his desire—have become sources of nourishment, sustainers of life for your baby.

Perhaps your husband's drop in desire didn't happen while you were pregnant or just after your baby was born; it happened as the kids got older. Watching you care for your children and become more and more immersed in the mother role has made it increasingly difficult for your husband to see you as a sexual being. He looks at you as "family," and for him, making love feels a little like committing incest. This change in his perspective does not have to be permanent, but until he discovers some way to grapple with it, it can diminish his desire for you.

LACK OF ATTRACTION

I can't tell you how many times someone in my practice has said, "I'm just not attracted to my spouse anymore," or "She's gained so much weight that I don't feel like making love," or "She doesn't care about how she looks. She's always in sweat pants at home," or "She used to work out all the time, and now she has let herself go," or "She never does anything to be sexually attractive. My feelings of attraction are gone now." But despite how frequently I hear these sorts of comments, feelings of attraction can be reignited. If your husband has said things like this to you, please don't despair, it's fixable.

Although it might seem unfair, unreasonable, unenlightened, or sexist, sexual attraction is a critical part of a sensual sexual relationship. Part of the reason for this is biology and evolution of human beings. Like other animals in the animal kingdom, we have distinct preferences for mates because we are all programmed for reproduction. Much of human sexual attractiveness is governed by physical attractiveness. Someone becomes physically attracted to another person based on that person's appearance, how he or she smells, and whether his or her voice is appealing. In a sense, we are hard-wired to be attracted to some people and not others.

So although your husband might really appreciate you for who you are as a person, his zest for you as a lover might disappear if you have changed physically in significant ways. Certain physical attributes cannot be improved. If this is true in your case, it will be best to get some professional help to see if you both can work around these issues. However, in the vast majority of cases, there are steps people can take to improve their physical attractiveness to their partners.

FEELING CRITICIZED

The more attention I paid to couples' problems with their sexual relationship, the more common it became to hear from men who completely shut down emotionally when they are criticized. In fact, criticism is likely to make a man feel "henpecked" or "castrated." Since a primary need for most men (and women) is to feel respected and appreciated by the women (men) in their lives, frequent criticism and put-downs often feel toxic. This prompts many men to completely avoid intimacy.

Are you critical of your husband? Do you feel free to comment on what you believe are his shortcomings? Do you find yourself noticing the things he does that irritate or disappoint you but fail to notice what he does right or the ways in which he tries to please you? Do you compliment him on a regular basis? Do your compliments outweigh your criticisms?

If, after thinking about these questions, you realize that your comments and actions might have played a part in causing the rift between you, that's a good thing. Once you realize that you've been pushing your husband away, you can change how you relate to him, especially if you know how much it is hurting him and affecting your sexual relationship.

UNRESOLVED FEELINGS OF
ANGER, RESENTMENT, OR HURT

When I talk publicly about low sexual desire, everyone immediately assumes I'm talking about women. When I say that I'm referring to men, people assume that it must be men who have physical problems such as erectile dysfunction. While erectile dysfunction is a major cause of low sexual desire in men, it's certainly not the only reason men turn off to sex. In fact, many men lose interest in sex for much the same reasons that women do: unresolved feelings of anger, resentment, hurt, and disappointment that make the idea of hopping in bed, kissing, and making love not very appealing. When women feel this way, we expect it, but we assume men want sex no matter what's going on in the relationship. So much for stereotypes!

I've seen many marriages where the women are the ones who want to be close physically after conflict. To them, it's a way of reconciling and re-connecting. These women can't understand why their husbands are keeping their distance because they feel certain that touch is a great healer. But try telling that to their men, who just want time alone to lick their wounds.

If you and your husband have been arguing a lot and he seems stand-offish, you just might have married a sensitive guy who needs to have everything in place emotionally before he can allow himself to be open with you physically. If this is the case in your marriage, good communication and conflict resolution skills will be the perfect aphrodisiac.

AVOIDING CONFLICT

Is your husband someone who broods about things but won't tell you when something is bothering him? Or he won't tell you what irks him when it's happening, but after a period of time, when he has about reached his limit, he explodes and lets it all hang out? If that's your guy, I can tell you a few things about your marriage.

First of all, you are probably shocked when he fires away at you because you don't see it coming. And even if his point has some validity, you feel convinced that the reaction seems out of whack and exaggerated com-pared to whatever you had done to set him off. And you're right; it is. Keeping anger and resentment inside in order to avoid conflict is an effec-tive way to mess up a marriage and kill any feelings of intimacy. This is not to say that your husband should call you on every little thing. Of course he shouldn't. But holding things inside separates people and allows anger, re-sentment, and hurt to percolate. Percolated negativity kills desire.

THE SEESAW PHENOMENON

Relationships are like seesaws: the more one person does, the less the other one will do. For example, the more one person cooks meals, the less the other even thinks about preparing food. The more one person expresses feelings, the more close-mouthed his or her spouse becomes. The more often one person sends out birthday cards to friends and relatives, the less the other one will assume that responsibility. And back to your favorite topic, the more one person wants sex, the less the other one will. So one of the reasons that your husband may be less than hot about sex at the moment might have something to do with the fact that you're thinking about it all the time. Right now, you have the job.

LOW SEXUAL IQ

Although the desire to have sex is instinctual, we're not born knowing how to be good lovers. We have to learn what it takes to turn on our spouses. And even if you or your husband have been previously married or have had other lovers in the past, what worked for that person may not work for your current partner. In short, we have to coach each other as to what we find stimulating and sensual. And to compound matters a bit more, because our bodies are always changing, what worked for us in our twenties won't necessarily work for us as we age.

What this all points to is the importance of having an open mind and being willing to learn more about sexually satisfying relationships. Even in the best of marriages, sexual boredom can set in.

> Before we were married, [my wife and I] had sex quite often and it was great! But then it got boring, and my wife didn't care. She only wanted to have it HER way (missionary, on top, or behind), which got old really fast! It wasn't very intimate; we never did anything else in the bedroom.
>
> Once, she took the initiative to do something different. I came home from work, and there were candles lit from the back door to the bedroom. There she was wearing the "sexy thing" I had gotten her for Christmas and she looked absolutely beautiful! I thought it was the beginning of a new chapter in our relationship. I was very excited and we started fooling around—something we hadn't done for a while. When there was a break in the action, she jumped up, looked at me, and said, "I can't believe I had to trick you into sleep-

ing with me!" I was speechless. I can't speak for all men, but I can tell you that if she stopped nagging me about sex all the time and started treating me more like a man, I would want to be more intimate.

There are many ways a couple can boost their sexual IQ. There are great books, DVDs, and sex therapists available; you'll find some of them listed in Chapter 13. But for now you should know that the key to boosting your sexual IQ lies in being open about learning new skills rather than becoming defensive when things aren't going well in the bedroom. Equally important is open communication with your partner. And therein lies the rub.

SEX TALK PHOBIA

It never ceases to amaze me how couples spend years and years together, raise children together, share a bathroom, see each other in the most naked of ways, and yet seem to be phobic about talking about sex. So many couples have confided in me that in all their years together, they have *never* talked to each other about their sexual needs, desires, fantasies, and fears. They don't tell each other what does or doesn't feel good. They don't say what they would like more or less of. They feel too embarrassed.

Maybe you are sitting here nodding your head in agreement as you read this. And if so, this might be one of the reasons your sex life isn't so hot. If you don't talk openly about sex, it may be hard to please each other sexually because you (or he) might be missing the mark. Even though we'd like people to be mind readers, they aren't. Your husband can't intuit what you find pleasurable, and you can't do this for him. So if sex hasn't been satisfying to him, he naturally wants to avoid it. If he thinks he's been unable to please you, he might stay clear of sex because he doesn't want to feel like a failure. Either way, if sharing openly hasn't been something you've been doing, it may explain your husband's sexual apathy.

LACK OF FORGIVENESS

Is your husband a grudge holder? Does he have difficulty letting go of past wrongdoings? Has something happened in your marriage that has deeply hurt or offended your husband? Has he told you that he has forgiven you, but it seems apparent that he hasn't really let the past be the past?

Or has your husband engaged in some behavior about which he has felt guilty or remorseful? Has he had an affair, and even though it's over, he can't quite seem to get back in step with you? Is your spouse a sensitive person who is hard on himself and has high expectations for his own behavior?

If any of these situations sounds familiar, your husband may be having a hard time forgiving you or letting up on himself. Either way, he is in pain. He might feel shame or grief about the past. He may even want to forgive and let go, but he doesn't quite know how. If this is true, the lack of forgiveness in his heart is making it challenging for him to feel close to you. Holding on to the past is not a good thing for anyone; it drains us emotionally, physically, and spiritually. A lack of forgiveness eats away at our immune system and puts us at risk of disease and other physical complications. People who are holding grudges have a hard time feeling joyful because they're stuck in the past.

If your husband fits this description, it is no surprise that he isn't approaching you sexually or being responsive to your sexual advances. Although moving beyond the past hurts, is hard work, and may take time, it can be done. I've seen it happen time and time again. Forgiveness can breathe new life into a marriage.

After reading the three chapters in Part II about why men say no to sex, you might be champing at the bit to turn over a new leaf and make things better between you and your man. The chapters in Part III will do just that.

~III~

Reaching Out:

The Solutions

~

CHAPTER SIX

What's a Woman to Do?

Before I begin sharing the steps you can take to improve things between you and your husband, I want to take a moment to congratulate you for having gotten this far in the book. You aren't just sitting around allowing your anger, resentment, or hurt to fester; you're doing something about your situation. You're willing to work hard to turn things around. So, kudos to you, girlfriend. You deserve a big pat on the back.

Since Chapters 7, 8, 9, and 10 are devoted to what you can do to improve your marriage and, in particular, your sexual relationship, I need to give you a heads-up: any time a woman tries to change a man, she should expect resistance. Generally men think of themselves as independent, self-sufficient beings and are really quite averse to being told what to do. Now, I know that you're not telling your husband what to do, but *he* might see it that way. Most men have radar for anything that even remotely feels like control and will resist it at any cost, even if what you're suggesting makes perfect sense and would beneficial to him. And when you heap on top of that the fact that you are addressing his sexuality, his ego might get extremely bruised, and if so, he will become defensive. I will help you approach your husband so that he will respond positively.

As you read the solutions in the following chapters, you need to know that there are no one-size-fits-all universal methods for boosting sexual desire. What works for one person might not work for another; it truly is a trial-and-error proposition. So don't get too bogged down trying to figure out the perfect place to start. Just start *somewhere*. If you are able to inspire your husband to try your suggestion and it proves helpful, keep going. If not, try something else. There will be plenty of ideas to choose from. If two or more solutions seem equally viable, that's okay. Again, it doesn't matter where you start, because a change in one area of your husband's life or your marriage will lead to changes in other areas as well.

In this chapter, I've outlined some general tips for influencing your husband. Take time to read them first because they will be helpful regardless of the route you choose. You will also read about the importance of setting solution-oriented goals. Ready for change? Great. Push up your sleeves, and let's get to work.

TIPS FOR GETTING THROUGH TO YOUR MAN

Be Loving

I know how much your husband's lack of interest in being sexual with you hurts and even angers you. However, if you approach him when you have anger in your heart, you will be transmitting those feelings. Even if you're not *saying* you're angry, he'll know. Before you approach your husband, you have to center yourself and come from a place of love and caring. Remember that no matter how upset you've been about all of this, he's been upset too. Even if sex isn't all that important to him right now, the fact that it's been such an issue between the two of you is wearing him down. Find some compassion, and take a deep breath before you speak to him.

Timing Is Everything

Regardless of what you wish to discuss with your husband, it's important to choose the right time. I know, there's never a right time to talk about this heated issue, but trust me on this one: some times are better than others. You might begin, "I have something important to talk to you about. Is now a good time?" If he says yes, then let 'er rip. If he growls no, ask him when he would prefer speaking with you. Then—assuming he doesn't respond, "In a decade," or something equally ridiculous—honor his suggestion.

Use "I-Messages"

One of the best ways to avoid defensiveness in others is to use "I-messages." If you've ever taken a communications skill-building class, you probably already know how to use I-messages. If so, remind yourself to use them when you approach your husband. It's easy to forget in the heat of the moment.

But since I don't know you, I will assume that you don't know what an I-message is. When you use I-messages, you talk about *your* thoughts and feelings rather than comment on what you believe your husband is thinking or feeling. Here's an example. Instead of saying, "I've asked you to read a book with me, and every time you say 'No,' you're just being controlling," you say, "I feel hurt when you turn down my suggestions to read a book together. It would really mean a lot to me for us to do this together." Or instead of saying, "Since you haven't gone to a doctor, it's clear that you don't care about my feelings," you say, "When you choose not to go to a doctor, I feel as if I'm not important to you." Talk about how *you* feel and avoid accusing, assuming, mind-reading, or diagnosing your husband. Then allow your husband to respond to your comments. He may not agree with your perspective, and that's okay. Feelings aren't right or wrong; they just are. Listen and acknowledge what you hear him say. For example, if he tells you that he won't read a book with you because he thinks that's a stupid idea, you might respond, "I know that you think reading a book together would be stupid, and maybe it would. But it's something I would really like to try." Don't become defensive or tell him he's wrong. Just continue sharing your feelings and your request.

Take Ownership of Your Feelings

Throughout your conversation, remember that regardless of how your husband responds, do not blame, criticize, or condemn him. You might even admit that you've been overly focused on sex recently because you've been missing him so much. Assume responsibility for what *you're* feeling rather than point to his inadequacies. Make sure he doesn't feel attacked. He needs to believe that you are on his side, no matter how challenging that might be.

Once you've set the tone for a collaborative, loving discussion, tell him that you realize that sex may be less important to him than it is to you, but you're asking that he take a step as a favor for you. Tell him why that would be such a good thing *for you*. Eventually he will see the benefit for him, but for now, he may not be able to see that. Don't let that deter you. Your husband doesn't have to agree that your sex life is unsatisfying or that the two of you have a major problem, and don't try to convince him of it. Just let him know that you will be the happiest person in the world when he does one thing for you.

Be Specific

Don't overwhelm him. Just ask that he do one thing, such as go to a doctor, initiate sex at least once a week, and so on. The more specific you can be, the better. Make action-oriented requests. For example, instead of saying, "I want you to care more about our sex life," say, "I got the name of a great doctor, and I'd like you to talk to him." Instead of saying, "I really need you to be willing to learn more about sex," say, "I heard about this seminar on low sexual desire that's being offered in town on Tuesday night. I'd really like you to attend it with me." Get the picture?

Find an Effective Hook

Talk to any talented salesperson, and she or he will tell you that no two buyers are alike and that in order to persuade someone to take action (buy), you need a hook. You have to find something that will motivate your "buyer" to "close the deal." For example, you wouldn't try to sell a home to a childless couple who plans on remaining childless by boasting about the quality of the school district. If instead what they were interested in was purchasing the home for investment purposes, a good salesperson would talk about how home values in the neighborhood continue to rise.

Similarly, when you approach your husband, you have to package your ideas in such a way that he feels inspired to change. You have to offer reasons that make sense to him. Along those lines, perhaps you've noticed that I keep suggesting that you take ownership for wanting a better sex life and stop trying to get him to agree that your sex life is a problem for him. I'm assuming that your husband might be more willing to change if he were doing it as a "favor" to you than if he thought he were flawed in some way. But the truth is, I don't know your husband, and that might not be an effective strategy. If not, you need to find some other hook that will inspire him to change.

For example, he might be more motivated to visit a doctor or take a positive step toward a better sexual relationship if it meant you would stop "nagging" him. I know you're not really nagging and that what you want from him is perfectly reasonable. But if he feels that you are nagging, he might be eager to do something different just to "get you off his back." Now, don't get your feathers ruffled. Remember, I'm on your side. But if you present it to him as a promise that you're going to stop nagging when he _____ (fill in the blank), he might be the first in line to do what you ask. If that wouldn't be a turn-on for your husband, just think about something that he'd find truly rewarding. Then package your request with a promise of your doing whatever floats his boat.

Reinforce Small Signs of Progress

If your husband shows *any* sign of coming toward you and agreeing to do what you are asking, such as saying, "I will think about it," or "I guess I can do that," thank him for his positive intention. Making a change always starts with thinking things through first. Few people just jump head-first into action. They have to mull it over for a while and get used to the idea that they are going to do something different. You can respond by saying, "Thanks, that sounds great. I will check in with you in a few days to see what you're thinking," or "Thanks for taking me seriously. I appreciate it very much. I have a great article for you to read while you're thinking things over."

HOW TO DEVELOP
SOLUTION-ORIENTED GOALS

Now that you have some ideas for getting through to your husband, it's time to set some goals. There's a saying that if you aim at nothing, you'll hit it every time—and it's true. So this section is about setting solution-oriented goals. Now I can just hear you say that you know your goal: you want your husband to stop moping around and start acting like he has a sexy wife, or something like that. That's not a solution-oriented goal. And if that's what you've been aiming at, no wonder you haven't gotten very far. Solution-oriented goals are goals that contain within them the seeds for solution, and I am going to help you become a master solution-oriented goal setter.

Here are three necessary criteria for developing solution-oriented goals:

Think About What You Want, Not What You're Unhappy About

When I ask people about their goals, they rarely tell me what they want. If I were to ask you what you're hoping to change about your marriage, you might say, "I wish my husband weren't so into himself and oblivious to me." Although this might make sense to you, you're focused on what makes you miserable, not what you want to see happen. A solution-oriented approach might be, "I would really like it if my husband paid more attention to me in the evening. I'd like it if he would flirt with me once in a while. All he has to do is to tell me I'm looking good, or he could grab my butt when I'm cooking." This response spells out what you want to have happen in your marriage as opposed to what you want to eliminate.

The problem with focusing on the things that make you miserable is that you're complaining rather than making a request for change. So instead of telling your husband, "I'm really unhappy about our lack of touching," you might say, "I love it when you kiss and hug me before we go to bed at night. That feels really good to me. I wish you'd do that more often."

Make Your Requests Action Oriented

When you say to your husband, "I wish you didn't ignore me when you come home," you're focusing on the problem. In addition, it's not clear exactly what you'd like your husband to do. No one is a mind reader, and you have to spell out in black-and-white terms what it is that you want and need.

An action-oriented requst is, "I would really appreciate it if you asked me to spend time with you in bed in the evenings. We don't necessarily have to make love; it would just be nice to snuggle once or twice a week." Here's another illustration.

Instead of saying, "Why can't you be more romantic?" you might say, "I would really like it if you asked me out on a sexy date once a month. You would agree to call the babysitter and find a new, romantic restaurant that we could try. I would also love getting e-mail from you once in a while. We used to have some hot exchanges, and it would be fun to get that e-mail again." Try it, and see what happens.

Go Slowly

Don't bite off more than you can chew. You need to break your ultimate goal down into steps—things your husband can accomplish within a week or so. Too many women ask for gigantic changes that might be reasonable but would take weeks, if not months, to carry out. By breaking goals down into small, doable chunks, success becomes more likely. And nothing breeds success like success. Here's an example:

Deanne felt that her husband, Vic, was incredibly inhibited when they made love. He would consent to be sexual only when the lights were off and if they made love in the missionary position. And no kissing, please. Since they had been married for over fifteen years, she felt that their love-making had become stale, and she was increasingly upset by this. When Deanne realized that she was starting to fantasize about another man at work, she knew it was time to do something constructive about her marriage, so she decided to confront Vic with her unhappiness.

Deanne told her husband that she wanted more variety and intimacy in their lovemaking. She clarified that by saying that she wanted to kiss him and take at least fifteen minutes for foreplay where they fondled and caressed each other. She also said that she had purchased new lingerie and wanted him to see her in it. This would necessitate keeping the light on.

Fortunately, Vic was open to hearing Deanne's requests and even shared some of his sexual hang-ups. So far, so good. But then Deanne told Vic that he didn't need to feel uncomfortable—that they could be experimental and try lots of new positions in the upcoming weeks. That's when their conversation headed downhill because Vic felt overwhelmed.

When Deanne had approached Vic, they were having sex once every two weeks at most; now it sounded to Vic that Deanne was going to initiate sex more frequently than usual. Plus, it appeared to him that she was going to insist that they experiment with novelty each and every time and that kissing—something they rarely had done together—was going to be a routine part of their lovemaking from then on.

While all this sounded great to Deanne (and probably you too), Vic got scared: although he was willing to change, it sounded like too much, too soon. Instead, it would have been helpful for Deanne to say, "Vic, I enjoy having sex with you. I would just like it to be a bit more creative. Here are some things we could do that will make a big difference to me [and list the action-oriented changes]. We don't have to do all of them at one time. Why don't we start off by agreeing to keep the lights on the next time we make love and start off with a few kisses?"

This approach sounds less threatening to a man who, for whatever reasons, is cautious in the bedroom. Ultimately he might need to talk to a therapist about his sexual inhibitions, but starting slowly is the best way to go, no matter what the problem.

And one more thing. When you're deciding what you're going to ask from your husband, make sure it's something he can do in a relatively short period, such as a week. Ask yourself, "What will be the very first sign that things are starting to be on the right track?" Accomplishing small steps is important because nothing breeds success like success.

In the chapters that follow, you will learn different approaches to boost your husband's sexual desire. It is my hope that you will find something to dramatically improve things between the two of you. Just think, you might be my very next success story! So read on.

CHAPTER SEVEN

Biological Solutions

There are so many biological conditions that could be affecting your husband's feelings about sex that if I were to attempt to educate you thoroughly about each possiblity, this book would be an encyclopedia. I don't have the expertise or time to write an encyclopedia, and you don't have time (or the interest, I presume) to read one. I am not a doctor; my expertise lies in helping couples resolve relationship issues. That's why most of my advice is geared toward helping you approach your husband differently in order to improve your sexual relationship.

Because getting a thorough checkup is a reasonable first step for anyone struggling with low desire, in this chapter I give suggestions on getting your man to a doctor. This chapter also offers information about biological treatments for testosterone deficiency and sexual dysfunctions because they are common reasons men lose desire. If you want more in-depth information about these subjects, check out Chapter 13, where I offer a helpful list of resources to further your education.

Your goal should be to pique his interest with enough information so he will want to know more.

Research tells us that a healthy and robust sex life has less to do with one's age than it does with physical health. If you want to remain in good health throughout your life span, you have to lead a healthy lifestyle. People who eat and sleep well; exercise regularly; avoid excessive alcohol, caffeine, or tobacco use; reduce stress through meditation, yoga, or biofeedback methods; build and maintain loving relationships; and screen for early detection of medical illnesses on a regular basis are likely to lead healthier, longer, and sexier lives. Anything your husband does toward maintaining a healthy lifestyle will go a long way to boosting his sexual desire.

But not everyone enjoys good health, and as I mentioned before, many underlying medical conditions interfere with sexual desire, including:

Heart and lung disease
Liver, kidney, and pituitary disease
Anemia
Parkinson's disease
Diabetes
Rheumatoid arthritis
Cancer
Thyroid disease
High blood pressure
Lupus

Low sexual desire is often the first sign that something is amiss; it could even be considered a blessing in disguise because it can alert a physician to a condition that requires medical attention. And the good news is that once your husband is successfully treated for an underlying medical condition, chances are that his desire for sex will return.

Common medicines, both prescription and over-the-counter, can also dampen your husband's desire. These include many antidepressants, tranquilizers and mood stabilizers, antacids, antibiotics, antiepileptic medication, antihistamines, anti-inflammatories, chemotherapy, and hypertension medications. A simple change in medications can often make a gigantic difference in how your husband feels about sex. For example, if your husband is on a popular antidepressant such as Zoloft, his desire level might plummet. Wellbutrin is an effective alternative drug that does not cause this problem.

Your husband may need a gentle nudge to seek medical advice, and in that case, you need to take charge. Even if your husband halfheartedly agrees to see a doctor, don't leave scheduling the appointment up to him.

Do it yourself, even if you think he should be more responsible. *Don't* do what this woman did.

> I haven't come right out and asked my husband to go to the doctor. I mentioned it a while back when he started having trouble with his erections. I told him that he shouldn't be ashamed to go. I also told him this could very well be physical and maybe something could be wrong health-wise. He has mentioned several times that he thinks he should go. He has also made comments like, "It is broke, I really need to get checked out." But then he will be out doing activities or be over at a friend's house when he very well could have made time for the doctor. The way I see it, is that it isn't a priority for him. This is building a whole lot of resentment in me. I don't feel like I should have to mother him and schedule him an appointment. Oftentimes I feel like the parent in this relationship. I am trying hard to break that trend.

The same is true for other goals you might have such as joining a health club, going out on a date together, or refilling a prescription. If he's willing to go along with your plan, register him at the health club, get the babysitter (even if you're the one who does it all the time), and pick up that prescription. Don't wait for him to do it. Don't keep score; get the ball of change rolling yourself. Want to know why?

I know a fifty-nine-year-old man who, when he finally told his wife that he had a problem, he *really* had a problem. He was bleeding rectally, and profusely. His wife insisted on rushing to the hospital. In the car, he confided that he had been bleeding for about a week. He had lost so much blood that once they got to the hospital, he needed two transfusions and was placed in intensive care. Yikes! What was this guy thinking?

Apparently he was thinking what many men think: "I don't need to go to a doctor. I will just tough this out." Bad decision. According to a Census Bureau survey, about a third of men report never seeing a doctor in a twelve-month period. Judging from the men in my practice, I would have to say that their doctor-phobic behavior is a lot more extreme than that. And when you take into consideration that a man has a fifty-fifty chance of developing cancer, that men typically die about five years before women, and that African American men die at least a decade earlier than white women, one would think a regular visit to the doctor would be a prudent thing to do.

Not only do men put off regular screening tests or intervention when there's an undiagnosed but recognized problem, surveys tell us that men who have been diagnosed with serious illnesses *still* avoid medical help. So if men avoid doctors, it should be no wonder that a man with low sexual desire would be resistant to scheduling an appointment with a physician. He's too busy convincing himself that a bad sex life isn't going to kill him. He feels mortified by the idea of talking to someone about a very, very personal problem.

Nonetheless, it's up to you to encourage him to get the help he needs. Research suggests that women are the ones to get their husbands medical attention. Single men or those who are widowed or divorced have significantly more health problems. Make that phone call for him if he's willing to go, and offer to accompany him if it would make him feel more comfortable.

If your husband already has a relationship with a family doctor, start there. Your husband may be referred to a urologist, endocrinologist, or even a sex therapist. Once your husband goes to his appointment, the doctor will probably ask questions about his medical history and any medications he might be taking. Additionally, the doctor might want to know about your husband's religious background, his past sexual relationships, and his current sexual relationship with you. The doctor will inquire about the onset of the problem, any discernible patterns, and concerns your husband might have about his life, including your marriage. Finally, the doctor might do a physical exam and order additional tests.

Let's look at some common problems and ways to deal with them.

LOW TESTOSTERONE

One of the reasons that so many medical conditions affect sex drive is that many illnesses drastically reduce levels of testosterone, one of the primary hormones responsible for sex drive. Besides losing interest in sex, a man with low levels of testosterone is likely to feel tired, have difficulty focusing or concentrating, and feel irritable or depressed.

If your doctor suspects that your husband's testosterone level is low, he will probably want to do a blood test. Because testosterone is usually highest in the early morning, testing is generally done at that time. The doctor will be particularly interested in your husband's levels of free testosterone (the amount of this hormone in his body that is available to do the necessary work). If it is in the low range and your husband has no underlying medical conditions that might worsen if testosterone is added (such as prostate cancer or sleep apnea), a testosterone supplement will probably be prescribed.

Men who take testosterone supplements often report an increase in energy, sexual desire, and fantasies, and a strengthening of erections and orgasms:

My husband's sex drive completely vanished after we got married, and it would be months in between having sex—and I think those times were more out of guilt on his part because I would get angry and we would fight about it. It was really tough for me to deal with, because I couldn't help but think that he wasn't attracted to me, that he didn't love me, etc. He kept reassuring me that it wasn't that. His standard answer was that he didn't know why and that things would get better. Things didn't get better, so I convinced him to see a counselor. After a number of sessions, she suggested that he have his testosterone levels tested.

Turns out he had hypogonadism—his body was producing extremely low levels of testosterone. My husband is only thirty, and we never thought of this. The remedy for him (and me) has been weekly injections of the hormone and the return to a good sex life. I can't believe how much better things are. I'm so glad I went to that counselor.

Testosterone supplements come in various forms—pills, gels, ointments, patches, creams, injections, and lozenges. The doctor can help your husband decide which method best fits his lifestyle. Patches containing testosterone can be applied to your husband's body; they release a steady level of the hormone that is absorbed through the skin. Gels are rubbed on various parts of the body, and the testosterone is absorbed through the skin. Some men get or self-administer injections every two weeks. It is also possible for your husband to dissolve a pellet containing testosterone under his tongue or against his gums. Oral testosterone is also an alternative, but experts are concerned about liver problems, high cholesterol, or heart disease when it is taken this way.

SEXUAL DYSFUNCTIONS

Primary male sexual dysfunctions are erectile dysfunction (ED), premature ejaculation (PE), and delayed ejaculation (DE). Although these dysfunctions often have biological *and* psychological causes, because the problem appears physically, I've included it in this chapter.

Erectile Dysfunction

Although my wife and I fooled around before we were married, we didn't have intercourse. I was nervous when we were making out and touching each other but I assumed that once we got married, sex would be smooth sailing. Unfortunately, saying the vows didn't take away all the fear and anxiety, and it sure didn't make us instantly proficient at sex. It was awkward, and we were confused, and I immediately started blaming myself. I thought that if there was a problem, it meant that I wasn't a real man. So although we figured out the mechanics of arousal and intercourse, we got a rocky start, and the anxiety would occasionally get the best of me.

This was before Viagra. It was also before a lot of the current therapy for erectile dysfunction. The anxiety was there to some degree most of the time. We would get into a good sexual rhythm, and then it would stop. My wife would get upset about it, and I would get things going again . . . for awhile, and then it would stop.

Now I understand that had I gotten treatment back then, we could have solved this problem years ago. In fact, the sex therapist we went to said that it was still possible that we could totally reverse this. But my wife walked out of the therapist's office mad and refused to continue counseling. She said we had nothing left: no friendship, no romance, and not even sex.

This story—filled with shame, hurt, and ignorance—is so sad. And the saddest part of all is that it is totally avoidable. I included this story because I want you to see that without guidance, sexual problems have the potential to destroy a relationship. It doesn't have to be that way. The best way to prevent ED is to encourage your husband to live a healthy lifestyle: limit his use of alcohol and other drugs, quit smoking, exercise on a regular basis, engage in routine stress- and anxiety-reducing activities, deal with underlying emotional issues such as depression, and aim for seven or eight hours of sleep every night.

But let's just say that your husband doesn't listen to your good advice and experiences more than just an occasional difficulty with getting or maintaining an erection (which, by way of reminder, is perfectly normal). What should you do?

Again start with a visit to the doctor. Women tell me that they have an easier time getting their husbands medical help when they suggest that their ED might be due to a physical problem. Apparently men feel less shame if they believe "it's not just in their heads." Here's a bit more information about biological treatments your husband might be offered to help him overcome ED.

Medications

You probably already know all about Viagra, the first oral medication available to men for ED. Newer drugs such as Levitra and Cialis, which have fewer side effects, are also available. These drugs increase blood flow to a man's penis and make sustained erections more likely. Viagra and Levitra work within about thirty to sixty minutes. Cialis generally takes thirty minutes, and the effects last longer. Studies suggest that these drugs work between 40 and 80 percent of the time with proper stimulation.

Although drugs like Viagra have vastly improved many couples' lives, it is unwise to rely solely on medication to improve your situation. You both need to learn more about ED and ways to build intimacy and emotional security, including excellent communication skills. Because relapse is common, couples who can talk about difficult issues have a much better chance of freeing themselves from ED permanently.

Although these medications have been a godsend for many, they are not always effective. Plus men with heart problems, stroke victims, or those taking nitrate medications should not take them.

Prostaglandin E is another drug used to help men with ED. It helps relax the muscle tissue in the penis, which, like Viagra, allows for more blood flow. This drug can be injected into the base or side of your husband's penis, which will produce an erection in five to twenty minutes; the erection will last for approximately one hour. The injection is said to be only minimally uncomfortable. This drug can also be used with a disposable applicator that inserts a small suppository into the tip of your husband's penis. Although this does not involve an injection, men often find the suppository method uncomfortable.

Vacuum Constriction Device

Another treatment option is an external vacuum device, a hollow plastic tube attached to a pump. Your husband will place the tube over his penis; the pump creates a vacuum, which causes blood to rush into his penis and causes an erection. Once he has an erection, your husband will slide a ring around the base of his penis; this will prevent the blood from exiting the penis and will maintain the erection. The vacuum and tube will be removed at this time. Your husband's erection will in all likelihood be maintained long enough for the two of you to have intercourse. After intercourse, the ring is taken off.

Vascular Surgery

A more invasive treatment, usually reserved for men who have experienced some sort of injury to the penis or pelvic area, is vascular surgery. An injury often blocks blood flow to the penis, making erections difficult or impossible. Surgery can sometimes correct this blockage. However, this surgery is considered experimental.

Surgical Penile Implants

Rigid or flexible rods are sometimes implanted in a man's penis to make it stand erect. There are inflatable versions that allow a man to inflate or deflate the rod at will. Although these prostheses do not create real erections, intercourse is possible. This surgery is not reversible and is considered a last-resort treatment for ED. As with any other surgery, there is a slight risk of complications.

Nonmedical Approaches

While it's true that there are medical solutions to ED, experts tend to agree that relying purely on medical solutions is shortsighted. For one thing, it makes ED all about your husband and his penis. That's unrealistic and nerve-wracking to boot—just what your husband doesn't need. You have a much better chance of really working through ED issues when you do it as a couple. So let's take a look at what you can do to help your husband with this issue.

I highly recommend that you start by reading Dr. Michael Metz and Dr. Barry McCarthy's book, *Coping with Erectile Dysfunction*. Although it is written for men coping with this issue, there is lots of good advice for their partners too. For instance, the authors allude to a common mistake women make when their husbands are coping with ED. In an attempt to be comforting, many women tell their husbands not to worry about their erectile problems—that intercourse really doesn't matter. If you have been telling your husband this, you need to reconsider this approach. I know you have the best of intentions but telling him you don't care about having intercourse (1) probably isn't true, and (2) you will be sending him an unsexy message; you will sound too motherly. Being indifferent about great intercourse isn't a very hot, juicy way to be. Despite his difficulty, your husband should have the feeling that having satisfying intercourse is something you very much desire and that you are willing to work with him to overcome this problem. Tell your husband that *until that happens,* you're eager to discover sexual activities you both find pleasurable and sensual and that lead to emotional intimacy.

While it may be difficult, it's important for you not to take your husband's ED personally. Chances are he's not having an affair, you're not unattractive, he's not mad at you, he hasn't fallen out of love with you . . . did

I forget anything? I know how easy it is for you to blame yourself for the situation, but you've got to get a grip on this. The more you dream up reasons this whole thing is your fault, the more you will question him. Questioning him, as I've pointed out before, will push him away because he feels bad enough about himself already. He is so wrapped up in self-doubt that he's unable to offer you any genuine reassurances. He's not feeling confident or comfortable, and he doesn't have it within himself to offer those things to you.

Additionally, if you continue to spend time ruminating about how this is your fault, eventually you'll become distant and disconnected. You will feel bad about yourself, and you will withdraw. The friendship and warmth will leach out of your marriage. You'll stop being physically affectionate; you'll quit touching each other and looking into each other's eyes. You'll stop laughing and talking about your lives together. And while this might build some protective armor around you, it won't feel very good because the pain will always be just below the surface.

Lisa and Devon had been married for five years. In the first year of their marriage, Devon would have difficulty staying hard once every few months or so. Lisa was very understanding about those times and reassured Devon that she enjoyed sex nonetheless. But over time, things got worse and Devon was experiencing difficulty several times a month. Lisa started to wonder if something was wrong.

Each time they made love and Devon faltered, Lisa asked questions. She asked whether Devon had lost his attraction for her, but he said that he hadn't. She wondered whether he was having an affair and if his inability to maintain his erections were due to any guilt he might be feeling. He denied any wrongdoing.

With each lost erection, Lisa began to ruminate as to the possible reasons he was not able to continue making love to her. The more she asked Devon about what was wrong, the more he felt interrogated. The more he felt interrogated, the more anxious he felt when they attempted to make love. The more anxious he felt . . . well, you can see where I'm headed with this.

What started out as a small problem ended up as a big problem because of the way in which Devon and Lisa tried to cope with their situation. Although Lisa's feelings of insecurity are understandable, she was inadvertently making things more uncomfortable for Devon.

So, how do you prevent yourself from asking constant questions or pulling a million miles away? It's all in what you tell yourself about this predicament. If you tell yourself that your mate is not attracted to or in love with you, you're setting yourself up for problems. If you tell yourself that he's out to hurt you or doesn't care about your feelings, you're bound to feel bad. Why not tell yourself something infinitely more constructive—something that will allow you to really be present for him as he struggles through this transitional period? Why not talk to yourself in ways that offer inner peace rather than constant turmoil? Try to replace your hurtful and destructive thoughts with more productive thoughts. Make them your mantras:

- I know we can work through this as a couple.
- I am not responsible for his erection. I can help, but ultimately we are each responsible for our own arousal and sexual satisfaction.
- This is not about me. I am a lovable and attractive partner.
- Although this is very hard on me because I miss him, he's hurting too, and I need to be emotionally available to him.
- There are skills we can learn together that will help us grow sexually, emotionally, and spiritually.

Another mistake I see women in my practice make when coping with ED is to go overboard in the opposite direction. They spend big bucks at Victoria's Secret, buy lots of sex toys and new perfumes, wear plunging necklines and short skirts, and amass big collections of sex-enhancing articles from women's magazines. In the bedroom, they up the ante by groaning louder, rubbing harder and longer, and swinging from chandeliers or installing stripper poles. This is all to no avail because ED is generally not about a man's inability to feel aroused. And, imagine the pressure your husband feels if you turn up the heat sexually.

I did everything to help him with his erectile dysfunction. I was caressing him any time I got the chance, telling him how sexy he is, licking the sweat off him, cuddling him, stroking him when he was hard, rubbing his nipples, stroking his body hair. You name it, I have done it. I've made porn films for him, got all the sexy underwear he asked for, complimented him. I kept myself up, wearing what he said he liked, however uncomfortable it was. He said all the right things, but he either went soft or went to sleep. Then HE felt like the victim when I broke down and cried. I am thinking this is unfixable.

So, what exactly can you do to help him? Plenty.

The first thing you need to do is an attitude check. Do you consider problems with erections or ejaculating *his* problem, or is it a couple's problem? The correct answer here is "a couple's problem." A sexual dysfunction is a couple's problem. It affects both of you and because you, as his sexual partner, are bound to have feelings about your husband's sexual challenges, the way you respond to the problem has a direct bearing on the outcome. Your response can have a positive effect or, as this man wrote, a not-so-positive one:

> As a man with a low sex drive, I can tell you it is a serious problem for the man. But it is so hard to talk about. When I try to talk to my wife, she gets mad. When I tell her it's not because of her, she refuses to believe me. And it's not her. Believe it or not, the problem is not always a lack of interest in the other person. Sometimes I really want to have sex, but if I worry about it too much, the chances of success drop dramatically.

This man's wife had little insight into the ways in which her anger and dismissal of her husband's feelings made things worse for him and their sexual relationship. The bottom line is that you need to work as a team on any sexual problem.

To help you take the sting out of your reaction to your husband's sexual difficulty, you need to recognize that men first learn about sex through masturbation, a highly predictable way to have sex. There is no other person to take into consideration, no one's feelings to gauge or responses to watch, no one to impress or let down. With masturbation, men don't have to "perform," and they don't have to connect. Success is easier to come by. (No pun intended.)

Sex with a partner, on the other hand, is an interactional experience that requires different skills. At its best, sex is not only about physical pleasure; it's also about intimacy and connection. Some men never quite master relationship skills, and when they don't, making love becomes an uphill battle. They feel frustrated and embarrassed. They never feel completely competent or good about themselves as men. And when they don't feel confident, sex can be an emotionally painful experience for them.

In addition, prior to age thirty-five, men's erections often happen spontaneously. Once they have to work at achieving erections or having successful intercourse, many panic. They think something is wrong with them when, in fact, nothing is. It's just nature taking its course.

Here's another interesting point. Research tells us that women are orgasmic approximately 70 percent of the time and don't consider nonorgasmic sexual encounters to be failures. But if a man fails to have an erection or ejaculates too quickly 30 percent of the time, it's likely that he or his wife will consider it problematic. So what's the solution? Become an erotic, loving friend to your husband. Ask him to share with you his story about times he feels most comfortable and confident sexually. Adopt a curious, noncritical stance, and listen in a way that allows him to feel safe to share what he's thinking. Let him know that ultimately, you are responsible for your own sexual satisfaction. He does not have to perform herculean feats to make you happy; you just want him to be your erotic mate, not a performer. You would like to share erotic and sensual pleasures with him. You want to play sexually. Remind him that sex is not a pass-fail subject. It's not about performance; it's about mutual physical, spiritual, and emotional enjoyment, and that's something you can experience together.

Premature Ejaculation

Premature ejaculation (PE) is men's number one sexual problem. As I discussed earlier, PE simply means that a man ejaculates more quickly than he wishes and before his partner has had an orgasm. Although this happens in most marriages from time to time, when it becomes a pattern, it can be very disappointing and frustrating to all involved. If coming too quickly is something your husband has been struggling with, how can you help?

At the risk of sounding like a broken record, try to get him to go to a doctor for a physical checkup. Although experts generally believe that PE is caused by emotional or relationship-oriented factors, inflammation of the prostate gland and spinal cord problems can also be at the root of this sexual difficulty. Eliminating biological causes is a logical first step.

Your second step is to see if you can influence your husband to go to a sex therapist or a marital therapist who is knowledgeable and skilled in sex therapy. Sexual dysfunctions are highly treatable with the right help. The American Association of Sexuality Educators, Counselors and Therapists has a list of qualified sex therapists in your area. (See Chapter 13 for how to get in touch.)

Besides seeking professional help, here are some things you can do on your own. It may be that one of the reasons your husband ejaculates too quickly is that he is overly excited. It may help to slow him down if he masturbates at least an hour or two before you have sex. The disadvantage of this approach is that he will not be training himself to gain control, and some men, particularly older men, need more recovery time between orgasms.

Another reason men ejaculate too quickly is performance anxiety. It is often the case that one incident of a speedy finish can get a guy wondering about himself, his staying power, and his ability to please his partner. If he spends too much time worrying about it, the next time he has sex, he will be wondering, "Am I going to come too fast this time too?" When people worry, their bodies release hormones that make relaxation and experiencing pleasure difficult. They more they worry, the more likely it is that they will experience difficulty. In a sense, it becomes a self-fulfilling prophecy. It's hard to get out of that loop once you've entered it, but it's definitely possible.

The sixty-four-thousand-dollar question is, "How do you help your husband relax?" Take the pressure off, that's how. If your husband feels pressured by needing to perform, eliminate the performance. Sex therapists often recommend that couples do exercises that are purely sensual, and they're not meant to result in intercourse. This relieves your husband of any "responsibilities." These exercises, developed by Masters and Johnson, are typically referred to as sensate focus.

Sensate Focus

Most people learn about sensate focus in a therapist's office, but you can try them (or your own version of them) at home. Although instructions often vary depending on the therapist and couple, I can give you the basic idea of these exercises, which is to become more aware of the sensations that you feel and what is pleasurable or not.

You and your husband should set aside about an hour to do stage 1 of sensate focus exercises. Send the kids to your mom's or the movies. Make your space comfy and inviting. You and your husband are going to take turns stroking and caressing each other's naked bodies. When you are the stroker, you should pay attention to what you are seeing and feeling, not what you think your partner wants you to do. As the "strokee," the goal is to be in the moment; just focus on what you are experiencing by being touched. The person being touched is allowed to voice pleasure or displeasure; otherwise, the exercises are designed to be done with little or no conversation. During the first few times that you do this, genitals and breasts are off-limits. Even if you or your husband feel aroused, the exercise should *not* culminate in your having sex. This is not meant to be foreplay. This exercise should be repeated several times before proceeding to the next stage.

Stage 2 of these exercises is similar to stage 1, although you are allowed to include touching of genitals and breasts. Start with nongenital body parts, and work your way slowly to genitals and breasts. Continue to pay close attention to the sensations you feel as opposed to trying to become aroused. Intercourse is still off-limits. Again, do this exercise on two or three separate occasions before proceeding to the next stage.

Stage 3 involves the two of you touching each other at the same time. The goal is to pay attention to what it feels like to touch and to be touched all at once. Again, no sex, please. Do this two or three times.

In the final stages of this exercise, you should begin with mutual touching. Then you can sit on top of your husband, and rub your genitals together but there is still no intercourse allowed.

I bet you're wondering, "When can we have intercourse?" At the next "meeting," you can do all of the above, only this time it's acceptable to have intercourse. If your husband feels the urge to ejaculate quickly upon entering you, stop, have him pull out, and wait. Start all over again.

Sensate focus exercise has proven effective with couples struggling with sexual dysfunctions. It refocuses you on sensation and sensuality without being goal driven. It's relaxing, pleasurable, and extremely therapeutic. If your husband won't go to a sex or marital therapist who is knowledgeable about this technique, you can act as his sex coach. Even if he's been reluctant to have sex, he might be in favor of doing this exercise because there's no opportunity to fail.

The Squeeze Technique

The squeeze technique was also developed by Masters and Johnson. When you use this technique, your husband will have the opportunity to practice feeling excited without ejaculating.

Begin foreplay—kiss and caress each other, and fondle your husband's penis until he feels like ejaculating. He should let you know when this is about to happen. Immediately squeeze his penis where the head of the penis meets the shaft. Hold the squeeze gently but firmly for ten to twenty seconds until he assures you that he no longer feels like ejaculating. Let go of his penis, and do not stimulate him for thirty seconds. Repeat this process several times so that your husband familiarizes himself with the feeling of being aroused but not ejaculating. After several repetitions, when he feels comfortable with this, you can have intercourse. If he feels overly aroused upon entering you, he should stop and withdraw his penis, and you can use the squeeze technique again. After several practice sessions, he will learn how to delay ejaculation without your needing to squeeze him. The good news is that 98 percent of men who become skilled using the squeeze technique learn how to successfully delay ejaculation. It's certainly worth doing. You can learn more about the squeeze technique in the suggested reading in Chapter 13.

Stop-Start Exercise

A more commonly prescribed exercise by sex therapists is the start-stop technique. The goal of this exercise is to help your husband become more aware of the sensations just before he ejaculates so that he can lengthen the amount of time he can maintain his erection while he feels stimulated.

Stimulate your husband's penis with your hand until he signals you to stop because he feels that ejaculation is imminent. You should then wait for about twenty to thirty seconds before stimulating him again. Have him tell you when he feels he's in control again. Do this several times. Your husband can also practice this himself through masturbation. In fact, the more he practices, the more control he is likely to achieve. In time, he will notice that he can be stimulated for longer periods before feeling the urge to ejaculate and that the time between stopping and starting becomes shorter in duration. In other words, he will have greater control. Once your husband feels more confident about his ability to control his ejaculation, the stop-start technique is practiced with intercourse.

Antidepressants

Forty percent of men taking antidepressants experience reduced sexual arousal. This is why doctors often prescribe these arousal-reducing antidepressants for treatment of PE! Zoloft, Paxil, Prozac, and some other antidepresants may help your husband delay ejaculation. Other kinds of antidepressants may also be effective in slowing your husband's ejaculation. It may not be necessary to take medication on an ongoing basis; simply taking a low dose before you plan on making love may be sufficient.

DELAYED EJACULATION (DE)

Delayed Ejaculation (DE), sometimes known as Retarded Ejaculation (RE) means that a man is unable to ejaculate or that it might take him thirty minutes or more to do so during intercourse. Couples who experience this during lovemaking often feel very frustrated. Some men are able to ejaculate more easily when masturbating, indicating that DE is not a physical problem. There can be medical causes of DE such as trauma to the pelvic nerves, certain medications, and medical conditions such as diabetes or high blood pressure, and excessive use of alcohol. Additionally, men who have had prostate surgery sometimes experience "dry" or retrograde ejaculations. During a dry ejaculation the ejaculatory fluid empties into the bladder rather than through the urethra. Nonetheless, DE is most typically caused by psychological issues such as anxiety, limiting religious beliefs, fears of pregnancy, discomfort with intimacy, and so on. If psychological issues are a concern, individual or couple therapy is recommended. Finally, sexual technique might be at the root of a DE difficulty. Sometimes the stimulation that occurs with intercourse is not sufficient for a man to achieve an ejaculation and couples need to be more creative in their love making. Sex therapy offers couples specific information about sexual practices that can eliminate the problem.

SEX OR MARITAL THERAPY

If marital issues are plaguing your husband and making it hard for him to relax in bed, a good marital therapist can help you to find effective and loving ways to deal with your differences. If your husband is dealing with personal issues from his past or from a current situation, he might benefit from individual therapy. The personal gains he will make from speaking to a professional might increase his confidence in lovemaking. A sex therapist can help both of you to learn skills to overcome sexual difficulties.

TELEPHONE COACHING

If your husband is too embarrassed to seek professional therapy, consider contacting a telephone coach through my office to overcome any relationship or sexual issues that still stand in the way of your having satisfying sexual encounters. The great thing about a telephone coach is the privacy and comfort it affords. I give contact information about my coaching program in Chapter 13.

CHAPTER EIGHT

Helping Him Deal
with His Issues

H as your husband been withdrawn, down in the dumps, or pre-occupied with issues that relate to his life and have little or nothing to do with you? Is he dealing with major job stress, or has he recently lost his job? Or are there other personal issues that are so consuming that he just isn't focused on you, your relationship, or your lives together? Or perhaps abusive childhood experiences have been preventing him from having a fully satisfying sex life with you. This chapter will help you generate some creative ways to help him overcome some of these troubling issues and get you and your sex life back on his radar screen.

When people are struggling with personal issues, they rarely have much to give to their loved ones. They feel overwhelmed, upset, depressed, confused, lost, or hurt, and it's hard to connect with other people. Some people use sex to boost their moods, but my guess is that your husband isn't one of them. Your husband is the guy who, when confronted with personal challenges, goes inside himself, and you become invisible. I want to remind you, first and foremost, that your husband isn't necessarily rejecting you personally, it's just that his emotional bank is empty. And when he's running on empty, he's not going to be approaching you for sex. In all likelihood, he's not going to be approaching you at all.

I know his self-absorption affects you and has a huge impact on your sex life, but again, it's probably *not* about you. Knowing this should make it a little easier for you to try to help him past his challenging times without so much self-doubt. He needs your help—but he might not be very receptive to accepting your help now. Sometimes people have to do things on their own timetables. Nonetheless, you might discover some new ideas that break through his stubborn resistance to change.

But understand this: When a person is struggling with a personal issue such as depression, poor body image, or unresolved childhood issues, you can't fix it for him. *He* has to want his life to be better. *He* will need to make the decision that he doesn't want to live with unhappiness anymore. So what can you do besides wait for him to see the light? Unless your husband gets professional help or puts a great deal of effort into using self-help resources, it will be difficult for him to free himself from his emotional discomfort. So, as with biological causes for low desire, you should start by encouraging your husband to get some professional help. You are not a therapist, and even if you are, you can't be your husband's mental health professional. It just doesn't work well that way.

Besides seeking professional help for any of these issues, there are steps you can take to get the ball rolling. *That* I will help you with.

Additionally, based on my long experience in working with couples, there are actions you should definitely avoid taking because, even with your good intentions, they can make matters worse.

DEPRESSION

If your spouse is depressed, you know firsthand how difficult it has been for him to lead a full life. You've also seen your sexual relationship go right out the window. A depressed person really isn't thinking about sex. In fact, 75 percent of people who are depressed confirm a loss of sexual desire. Regardless of the cause of your husband's, I know you've been hurt and frustrated by his emotional and physical withdrawal. You probably have had a hard time understanding why he doesn't just snap out of it.

Depression needs to be treated—your marriage and your sex life depend on it. With this in mind, your goal should be to convince your husband to do something about feeling crappy. It's challenging because most men don't like to admit they're feeling depressed. They feel vulnerable, and that's just unacceptable to them. But whether he admits it or not, you should be aware of the signs. Although I discussed the symptoms of depression earlier, they are worth repeating. Your husband might be depressed if he:

> Loses interest in sex
> Withdraws and says very little
> Seems unmotivated
> Is fatigued
> Gets angry a great deal
> Sleeps too much or too little
> Eats too much or too little
> Cries or frequently seems irritable
> Abuses alcohol or other drugs
> Seems anxious
> Feels worthless
> Has suicidal thoughts
> Loses interest in people

In addition, many men who are depressed complain about physical symptoms such as headaches, stomach problems, body aches, and pains. It's a lot easier for men to talk about physical ailments than to admit they're struggling emotionally.

Though you can't be his therapist, you *can* do some things that can increase the likelihood that he'll get help or will be more receptive to you in general.

Start with a Simple, Straightforward Approach

Approach your husband when he is not otherwise occupied, and tell him that you want to discuss something with him. Let him know that you are truly concerned about him. Discuss the signs you've been seeing in his behavior that have caused you concern. Give specific examples, such as, "You're usually so outgoing and interested in doing things with the family. Lately you've just been keeping to yourself," or "Throughout our marriage, you've always been physically affectionate. You haven't touched me for six weeks now. You seem really down." Or, "Generally, you are so patient with the kids. You've been very, very irritable lately, and I know that's not the real you." Or, "I know you like a glass of wine with dinner, but lately you've been drinking five or six glasses of wine and falling asleep on the couch. I can only assume that you're not feeling great or you wouldn't be doing that."

After expressing your specific concern, tell him that there are things he can do to feel better and, if he would like, you are willing to help him in any way you can.

Watch Your Language

You need to be careful of the words you use when referring to his depression. Even though you and I know he's depressed, that word can carry negative connotations in his mind. He might admit he's feeling down in the dumps, bummed out, or stressed out, but watch him recoil if you mention the "d" word. So, don't press it. Talk about his being "in a rut." You see, if he agrees that he's in a rut, he will need to do many of the same things to lift himself out of the rut that he would to free himself from the grips of depression. So, don't haggle about the term he uses to describe how he's feeling. If your husband still disagrees with your perception of him, ask if he will see a doctor or therapist anyway—just to sort things out. As long as you can convince him to be proactive in doing something to feel better, that's all that counts.

Congratulate Him on His Openness

If your husband is receptive to anything that you're suggesting, give him lots of kudos. Tell him you understand how hard it must be for him to acknowledge that he hasn't been feeling well. Remind him that it takes a strong man to admit that he has to work on something. Thank him for listening to you. This will be your opportunity to share your ideas about what he might do. Here are some suggestions to offer him:

- Get a complete medical/physical to rule out biological causes.
- Begin therapy with a goal-oriented therapist. Research tells us that depression is best treated by either talk therapy or a combination of talk therapy and medication. A family doctor and a psychiatrist can prescribe medication, but these professionals generally do not offer

help with the issues about which your husband might be depressed. A good therapist can help your husband work through emotional issues that are weighing him down. Make sure the therapist adheres to a goal-oriented, skill-building therapy model such as solution-oriented, cognitive, behavioral therapy rather than one that is focused on analyzing the cause of the depression. These therapy models will offer your husband tools for breaking free from depression in a shorter period of time.

• Meet with a psychiatrist or family doctor to assess the need for antidepressant medication. There are many different medications available that are effective in dealing with depression. No two people react the same way to specific antidepressants. Some people experience few or no side effects, whereas others are much more troubled by them. Frequently, a trial-and-error process is necessary to discover the best medication for a particular individual. Medications should be monitored by a physician. Also, remember that some antidepressants dampen sexual desire and arousal. If your husband is going to take an antidepressant, insist that he talk to his doctor about using one that won't complicate your sexual situation. And finally, know that antidepressants may take several weeks to be effective.

Respect His Ideas About Treatment

As you share your opinions about how to tackle your husband's depression, notice how he's responding to you. If he seems to agree that he's been feeling bad but has different ideas of what might help, don't debate him. As long as he gets his feet moving, you will both be better off.

Don't Be Defensive

It's possible that your husband will agree that he's depressed but he claims that *you* are the reason for his bad mood. And what if he offers you lots of examples of how you are pulling him down? It may be true that you have some relationship issues to work out, but at this point your husband is having a difficult time recognizing how his distorted thinking is playing a big part in the problem. Whatever you do, don't become defensive. If you defend yourself, he will have to go the extra mile to prove you wrong. He will scan his memory for all the bad things you've done recently and in the past that have created his sullen moods. I want to reassure you: research shows that a person's current mood state greatly colors his memory. If you ask depressed people about their lives, they tend to remember depressing events. Happy people, asked the same question, tend to remember happy events.

When your husband blames you for his misery and therefore for his lack of interest in sex, you might be asking yourself, "What! Is he nuts?" Please keep that thought to yourself. In fact, if your husband insists that your behavior is making him unhappy, even if you wholeheartedly disagree, offer to go to therapy with him. Tell him that you are willing to do whatever it takes to help him feel better. The point is that, regardless of the reason he's seeking help, he will be pointed in the right direction.

Look, I know that my suggestions require an enormous amount of self-control. You have to feel good about yourself to resist the temptation to volley with him if he says negative things about you. It's also important to avoid allowing your husband's depression-prompted comments to define you. You need to develop a Zen-like detachment from the things he says to you and his bad moods. Although this can be difficult, there are some ways you can help yourself stay centered.

For one thing, you need to be kind and loving to yourself and do things that feed your soul. You must have other outlets besides your husband for emotional support. Connect with people who love you and understand your situation. Don't hang out with people who say, "Why in the world would you want to put up with a husband who is depressed all the time and doesn't want to have sex?" If these "protective" folks are good friends of yours, tell them, "I appreciate your caring, but I want to make my marriage work." Then stop complaining about your spouse to them; their feedback won't be helpful to you. Find friends who have weathered similar experiences, and hang out with them. If you wait out the storm, your husband will see the light of day. That's when you'll realize the wait was well worth it.

Be Patient

Whether your husband is willing to get help or not, the one thing you will need to be is patient. Unlike a cold, which might lift in a few days, being depression-free takes time. In fact, even under the best of circumstances, people start feeling better little by little, but with many ups and downs along the way. Often when they begin to recover, they feel so relieved to be feeling better that the next bad day (which we all have from time to time) sends them into a tailspin. You need to know that your husband's recovery will be gradual, as will the return of his sex drive. Positive change rarely happens as quickly as we would like.

The Back Door Approach
Let's assume that your husband is not receptive to seeking professional help. Then what? I say you use the back door approach. This means that you encourage your husband to engage in depression-busting behavior without calling it such. Here is a list of things you can encourage him to do.

Exercise Aerobically
Research has shown that regular exercise guards against and alleviates depression. Among countless other health benefits, strenuous aerobic exercise stimulates the release of endorphins, the body's natural opiate. This will also help him feel better about his body, which may in turn help him feel more turned on.

Follow a Healthy Diet
A well-balanced diet ensures a healthy body, which is nature's best defense against the stressful symptoms of depression. And there are other things you should know about the role of diet and depression. For example, when blood sugar is low, mood swings are likely. Slow-acting or low-glycemic carbohydrates, along with high-quality fats and proteins, are believed to stabilize blood sugar levels and therefore are considered valuable resources for combating depression. Additionally, it is believed that omega-3 fatty acids, especially from fish or fortified eggs, are important depression busters. Consider consulting with a nutritionist or naturopath to help design a depression-fighting eating plan.

Explore Alternative Health Approaches
There are many alternative methods for dealing with milder forms of depression, such as supplements, herbal therapy, acupuncture, yoga, and meditation. These approaches do not require a doctor's prescription. In

states where acupuncture is licensed and regulated, you can get the names of practitioners by calling the state department of health or the department of licensing. Just make sure that the acupuncturist is board certified.

Additionally, you could encourage your husband to use B vitamins, particularly B_6, often referred to as the stress vitamins, vitamin C, supplements of DL-phenylalanine, the herb St. John's wort, or SAMe. Research suggests that the omega-3 fatty acids found in fish oil may be helpful in warding off depression. If your husband is taking any medication, you need to ask your doctor about possible interactions with supplements or herbs.

Focus on the Exceptions

Even while you're waiting for your husband to get help or benefit from the help he is receiving, you can do something about your sexual relationship by focusing on the exceptions:

If your husband's feeling down has affected his sexual desire, you are probably seeing things through that all-or-nothing lens. You believe that he never feels sexual, and maybe he doesn't. But there probably *are* times when he has been a bit more amorous. Recall the last time your husband was sexual in any way and ask yourself:

> "What was different about that time?"
> "What was I doing differently?"
> "What was he doing differently?"
> "What was different about our life at that time?"

See if you can spot any differences between the times he shows some interest in being physically intimate as compared to the times he doesn't. Here's an example.

Jennifer and George had been married for seventeen years and had two children. George had bouts of depression throughout their marriage, and during those times their sex life generally deteriorated. Jennifer and George assumed that depression was going to be a part of their lives because George's father had been prone to depression as well.

When Jennifer first learned about George's tendency to become depressed from time to time, she was very understanding and gave him the space she believed he needed. But recently, his bouts of depression had become longer, and his desire to interact with her and their children had become severely limited. During his most recent bout with depression, which had lasted six months, she told me, "George hasn't even come near me. Not once."

"I know George has been feeling miserable and that when he feels that way, he's likely to pull away from you," I said to Jennifer, "but I wonder if you could think about the last six months very carefully and recall a time when George was more present emotionally and maybe even physically too." Jennifer thought about my question for a few moments and restated that they hadn't made love for six months. George interrupted her and said, "That's not true. You and I had sex a few days after you visited your mother in Texas." I asked about the purpose of her trip. Jennifer replied,

My mother had some very serious health issues, and I went to help her. My father passed away five years ago, and she has no one else to give her a hand. When I was in Texas, George not only took over and handled the kids himself; when I got back he was very kind to me. I was pretty upset, having to be the only person willing to take out time to help my mom, and George was very understanding. I cried when I came home, and George comforted me. That led to our having sex, and it felt very good. That was four months ago, but he's right. It did happen.

I asked Jennifer and George to offer their best guess as to why George reacted as he had to Jennifer when she returned from Texas. Jennifer spoke first:

I never really thought about it, but now that you ask, it was kind of different. For one thing, I had been away for about a week. I am usually Super Mom, and George knows that I handle everything. That week George just had to step up to the plate and be the dad all by himself. He did a great job, and the kids thought so too. So I guess focusing on the kids took him out of his head and forced him not to obsess about things as much as he usually does. Maybe he missed me too! Who knows? I'd like to think that was true.

George replied:

You know, I felt sorry for Jennifer. She has two sisters, but they're selfish. They won't lift a finger when it comes to their mom. Jennifer is her mom's saving grace. I know it was hard for Jennifer to sort through the medical advice they had gotten from various doctors and to see her mom in pain. I just felt sorry that she had to be doing that alone.

"How is that different for you, George?" I asked. And he said:

When I'm depressed, I don't think about anyone else. I just curl up into a ball and think about myself and how my life isn't going well. I let Jen handle things, just like my dad did with my mom. And I guess, the more I am out of the loop, the more depressed I get. And when I feel that way, I definitely don't feel sexy, and I don't take Jennifer's feelings into account. I figure she can take care of herself. She's pretty darn independent. So what's different is that I felt needed. And she's right: I missed her. I love the kids, but being with them all week was hard. I appreciated what she does, and it got me out of myself. Plus, when she got home, I could tell she was tired and sad, and I know how that feels. So I wanted to comfort her. I don't usually get the feeling that she needs me to take care of her. I'm the "sick" guy, you know.

Jennifer was really touched by George's caring. She always knew that deep down inside, he loved her, but his increased distance made her question those feelings. She cried as he spoke of his concern for her.

I wanted to make sure that George and Jennifer understood why good things happened after her return from Texas. I wanted them to become skilled solution detectives, to extrapolate the learning lessons from their last lovemaking. Here's what we learned:

- George needs to be busy, even if he doesn't feel like it, because it takes his mind off his problems.
- George needs to feel needed and important in the family.

- For the sake of the kids and for their marriage, Jennifer needs to quit being Super Mom and insist George participate in the family. Without realizing it, Jennifer's inadvertently letting George off the hook wasn't helping George's emotional well-being.
- Jennifer needed to do more things for herself, away from their home so that George could both assume responsibility and miss her.

George and Jennifer learned something else as we discussed the exception. Jennifer realized how easy it was for her to overlook that small but important event. Could it be that, because of her past experience with George's depression, Jennifer had come to expect a sexless, affectionless marriage, and that was what she was noticing about their interactions? I couldn't help but wonder whether over the course of the six months, there had been other signs, even small ones, that George had been more affectionate despite his depression. Jennifer was intrigued by this possibility and agreed to give it more thought over the next few weeks. Additionally, she agreed to be more effusive with compliments when she noticed George getting outside himself and being more in the world.

George felt encouraged by our conversation because for the first time in a long time, he realized that he had some control over his mood. Even though he wasn't in the mood to take over the kids when Jennifer left town, he was able to do it, and the activity altered how he was feeling. Now he wondered about other ways he could consciously decide to take action that would improve his mood. That was new for George, and he felt optimistic about the possibilities.

In the remaining weeks of our work together, Jennifer and George applied what they had learned in our sessions. George's mood lifted significantly. He joined a health club and started working out regularly (even if he didn't feel like it). And instead of rocking in the dark when he was feeling down, he forced himself to stay with the family and do the best he could to interact with them. This boosted his self-esteem and his outlook in general. He found himself being more talkative and attentive to Jennifer. Although sex wasn't yet as frequent as Jennifer wished, they began making love again and being considerably more physically affectionate.

Focusing on one exception revealed an avalanche of relationship solutions for Jennifer and George.

POOR BODY IMAGE

One of the reasons your husband may turn off to sex is that he doesn't feel good about his body: his belly protrudes, his ass is huge, he hates his thighs, his penis is too small, he doesn't think he's muscular enough, he has flabby underarms, he's got too much hair (or not enough hair), and his acne is really getting the best of him. Show me a man with a poor body image, and I'll show you a man who doesn't like himself very much and certainly doesn't feel very manly. This can spell disaster for a couple's sexual relationship, but there are some things you can do.

Focus on the Positive, and Compliment Him

The first and most obvious step for you is to try to boost his ego by telling him what you like about his body. He might not be happy about the extra fifteen pounds, but you might like how strong and solid he feels. You may love the way he licks you or uses his hands on your body. You may adore the way he smells or the touch of his hair. Tell him what feels good about his body to you and what you love about his sexuality. See if your positive feelings can override his negative self-talk. Sometimes this works, and sometimes it doesn't. Negative self-talk can be quite compelling.

Don't Criticize or Nag

If your husband dislikes his body but isn't doing anything to become more fit, you might find yourself commenting or criticizing every time he grabs for the potato chips or ice cream. You may also notice that you're constantly cutting out articles or getting pamphlets about the local fitness gyms. In other words, you're a perpetual nudge. And while I totally understand that you're trying to help him feel better about himself, if your reminders haven't been working, you need to stop what you're doing. You're doing more of the same.

Catch Him in the Act of Getting It Right

If your spouse has a relatively unhealthful lifestyle, catch him in the act of getting it right, eating well, exercising, or being mindful about his health in any way, and let him know how great it is that he's making good choices. Don't belabor the point or go overboard, which might seem patronizing; just throw a compliment at him and stop. Remember that positive reinforcement is a powerful means of behavioral change.

Identify the Bigger Issue

Sometimes the key to low sexual desire induced by poor body image is not the obvious. It's not about discussing eating or exercising habits or even focusing on what's going on (or not going on) in your sex life. It's about discovering the underlying reasons a man isn't taking better care of his body and then addressing those reasons head-on.

Susie and her husband, Clay, were married for seventeen years. Susie is a registered nurse, and Clay is a school administrator. Their marriage was a good one until approximately five years ago, when Clay's mother died. Clay was very close to his mother, and her passing really took a toll on him emotionally. Although he had always led a very active lifestyle it all stopped shortly after his mother's passing. He also began to eat excessively when he felt overwhelmed with grief. It wasn't long before he gained twenty-five pounds and often felt fatigued. Clay frequently made derogatory remarks about his physique and his lack of muscle tone. He felt ashamed that he wasn't taking better care of himself physically. He completely stopped initiating sex with Susie.

Susie felt hurt and confused by his rejection and tried to discuss his feelings with him. Clay admitted that his lack of interest in sex was all about his not feeling manly or sexual because his body was so out of shape. As any other good wife would, Susie tried to reassure him that he was still attractive to her and that she was very much interested in making love nonetheless. Although in the past Clay had usually initiated sex, Susie took over his role and often became sexual with him, fondling his penis, offering massages, giving him gentle, sensual kisses, dressing up in new lingerie, and "talking dirty" to him. But according to her, none of this made any difference. Clay didn't want Susie touching him and pulled back from any affection for fear it would lead to something sexual.

After seven months of feeling put off, Susie came to therapy by herself. After learning more about their situation, I helped Susie to realize that Clay was still mourning his mother's death and that his sadness was what triggered his lethargy and self-neglect. Rather than address their sexual relationship head-on or his physically unhealthy choices, I thought that if Clay could begin to address his lingering sadness about his loss, he would feel better and would be more likely to engage in better self-care.

Susie needed to broach this sensitive subject with Clay, who hadn't discussed his mother's death for months. I coached her to tell him, "You haven't said anything about your mom for a long time, and I know you must be missing her. What have you been thinking about? What are you feeling about not having your mom around us anymore?" If Clay was willing to discuss his feelings, I suggested that she just listen, acknowledge his feelings, and show curiosity for learning more about his inner thoughts. She didn't need to have answers or guide him in any way; she just needed to be a loving friend and listen. Susie agreed to give this a try.

Two weeks later, Susie returned. She told me that Clay was not exactly open to talking with her the first time she approached him. However, she decided to try again later in the week, and he was responsive. Not exactly an expressive man, Clay had some difficulty talking about what he'd been feeling for so long. But Susie was patient, and her patience eventually paid off. Clay talked about his pain and his longing for his mother. He reminisced about many pleasant childhood memories. He laughed, he cried. They cried and hugged. Susie concluded their talk by reminding him that she was there for him, that he could talk with her about his feelings anytime. He thanked her for her caring.

In the days that followed, Susie noticed that Clay seemed more upbeat. Without saying anything about it, she went out of her way to make healthful dinners for them and invited him on walks with her. Because he was feeling better emotionally, he agreed. And although there had been no major weight loss in the two-week period between therapy sessions, Clay had become visibly happier. Right before our second session, Susie risked initiating sex with Clay when they went to bed one night, and Clay responded positively. Susie was delighted.

The moral of this story? If your husband feels bad about his body and is not taking the necessary steps to improve things, try to get a handle on the emotional issues standing in the way of his being good to himself. Focus on those issues in a loving way rather than discuss your sexual relationship or his health habits. Your caring and friendship might unleash a desire in him for the self-improvement necessary to be your sexual partner again.

STRESS

You've had it. Your husband has no interest in sex, and he tells you it's because he's too stressed out. He complains of working long hours, having too much responsibility at home, feeling overwhelmed by the kids, and hassled by you when you complain. You can see that he has a very short fuse. It's amazing that you even desire him because he seems so on edge all of the time. Sound familiar? What should you do?

You have a lot of options. You may be familiar with some of the ones listed here. If you do, breeze through them, and focus on the ones that sound more enlightening.

Begin with Prevention

At the risk of repeating myself . . . the best way to ward off stress is by doing the obvious things: eating well; exercising; getting seven or eight hours of sleep every night; avoiding excessive alcohol, tobacco, and other drugs; creating balance between work and play, being alone and socializing; and engaging in stress-reducing activities such as yoga and meditation. If your husband is frazzled and he's not doing much of the above, it's time to help him get his ducks in a row. Encourage him to take care of himself, even if it means some time away from you. A couple of hours at a health club will be a great investment in terms of his ego, mood, and sense of replenishment. He'll come back a better and maybe more willing partner.

Ask What You Can Do to Help

Sit down with your husband to discuss why he feels pressured and what you can do to help. There may be some things about his situation that are unchangeable, but if you put your heads together, you might discover some creative ways to make life feel a bit more relaxing to him. You might not like his suggestion or even agree that your doing it would help, but when he talks, you should listen. Don't be reactive; just hear him out. If he tells you, "I hate when I come home and the first thing you do is complain about the kids or how your day went," or, "I can't stand being at home when the house is cluttered," don't jump down his throat, even if you have a full-time job. Listen to his concern, and feed back to him in your own words what you heard him say. If you are comfortable with his request, let him know that you will do it. If you aren't so sure, tell him you heard him and that you will take his request to heart. Don't debate him about his feelings.

If your spouse has a hard time thinking of things that you might do that would be helpful, make some suggestions, and see if he thinks they might help. Even if you think he's overreacting or exaggerating, keep your feelings to yourself for now. Your goal is to help him feel heard.

Apply What You've Learned About Solution-Oriented Goal Setting

You will very quickly discover that your husband is much more likely to complain than he is to offer you constructive ideas about what he'd like to change to make life less stressful. You need to help him translate his complaints into positively stated action-oriented steps you both can take to lighten his load.

Step 1 is to help him describe what he wants as opposed to what he's unhappy about. When he tells you, "I hate when I come home and the first thing you do is complain about the kids or how your day went," tell him that you understand how stressful it is for him to hear your complaints as soon as he walks through the door. Then ask, "How would you like things to be different? What would help?" Hopefully, he will say something like, "It would really be nice if you could just give me fifteen minutes to unwind before you tell me anything about the kids or about what went wrong that day," or "Instead of starting the evening with a litany of complaints, could you just say one thing that went well at home?"

Step 2 is to help him identify action-oriented goals. Most people are far too vague when they think about what they want to change in their lives. If he tells you, "I can't stand being at home when the house is cluttered," ask, "What would need to be different for you to feel more at peace at home?" Your goal is to have him define *specific* actions such as, "All I really want is for the toys to be picked up and for your magazines to be put out of sight rather than in piles all over the house."

Step 3 is to make sure he is asking you for something you can do in a relatively short period of time. I once worked with a couple who had completely opposite needs for order in their home. She was a packrat, and he was the world's tidiest man. He grew increasingly resentful about the collections around the house and withdrew emotionally from his wife. They stopped having sex.

When I discovered that this tidiness issue was at the heart of their passion problem, I asked him what would need to happen for him to feel less resentful and more connected to his wife. He spent the next ten minutes describing a long, long list of home improvement to-do's. I stopped him and said, "You know, I can really understand that you want these projects to happen and you want them now, but your cluttered house took a long time to get that way, and it isn't going to change completely overnight. So, tell me, what would your wife have to do that would signal to you that she is serious about tackling these projects and caring about your feelings? What would be at the very top of your to-do list?" This man itemized a couple of small but important clean-up tasks that were doable in a week's time. His wife seemed relieved and accomplished those goals. He felt heard, appreciated, and warmer toward her. Then, surprise, surprise, they were more physically affectionate.

Don't Overlook the Bigger Picture

I want to address the importance of keeping an eye on the bigger picture. I recently coached a man who was trying to save his dying marriage. He told me that he had had a persistent headache for five years. He traveled the country going to specialists but no doctor could find what was causing these nagging headaches.

I found that strange, because you really didn't need a medical degree to understand why this man's head was pounding. He had an extremely high-pressured career, worked seventy to eighty hours a week, his wife felt neglected, his children were hyperactive when he finally returned home, and he had a short fuse to boot. Because he had to "get it right every time" at work, when he got home he just wanted to veg out, not be sociable, and not do much of anything at all. His wife grew steadily weary of his behavior and lack of involvement with their family and social life, but he still showed up for work every day, day after day, for ten years. Let's see, can you think of a reason this man might have had a headache?

At some point, when a person feels so stressed that nothing feels pleasurable or relaxed, it may be time for a serious look about what needs to change. It may not be as simple as keeping the kids calm or having a warm dinner ready when he comes home. Your lifestyle may need a major overhaul. So while you're looking at specifics, don't overlook the bigger picture.

Remember to Touch

If your husband feels that there is too much on his plate and he's feeling frazzled, the last thing he is going to want to have is another responsibility. And if he feels that he has to "perform" for you or go to great lengths to satisfy you, it may just put him over the edge. Tell him that you'd like to relax with him and give him a massage or just cuddle with each other. Tell him that it's not intercourse that you're after; he doesn't need to give you an orgasm and satisfy you sexually. You just want to help him to unwind. You never know what might happen.

Timing Is Important

I've said earlier in the book that men's testosterone level is highest in the morning, So why wait until the evening when he's tired, overworked, and overwhelmed to approach him sexually? He may feel more rested and horny just after he wakes up. Pay attention to his calmer, sexier times, and take advantage of them.

GRIEF

Change and loss are inevitable, and grief is a normal response to loss. The larger the loss, the greater the grief.

Someone who is grieving is often consumed with sadness. Little else matters. Thoughts about the impact of the loss or past memories are played over and over in the mind of the grieving person. Concentration on daily matters becomes challenging. Those who grieve also often feel guilt, remorse, and anxiety. They frequently avoid socializing or interacting with others. Many seem angry or irritable. As with depression, grief can result in physical symptoms such as fatigue, changes in sleeping and eating patterns, and a total disinterest in sex.

> I've lived with the same man for almost twenty years, and for the last ten, we've had virtually zero sex life. Not only sex, but our marriage has also been void of affection, intimacy, and maybe love . . . He is not interested in finding out what, if anything, is wrong. We were in therapy for about three sessions last winter, up until the therapist suggested he have a hormone test. That was the end of that.
>
> He shows pretty much zero interest in me, will not come near me, backs off whenever I'm near him, and cannot on any level talk about sex or sexuality. I've thought of many ways to have an affair, but have not taken that route. Why, I really don't know. Up until recently, I thought and felt that I still loved this man, but I'm beginning to wonder why I am spending the best years of my life with someone who clearly thinks I'm disposable.
>
> I should have prefaced this by saying that our relationship took a huge detour in 1996 after his younger brother died of AIDS. It seemed to kill a part of him, and for a long time, he walked around blaming me and telling me how he didn't give a damn about me or anything. I had faith this would change, but it didn't. My life seems dark and dreary most of the time. It is a hard road to walk. I have never read or heard people talk about living like this. I kept waiting for that man who wanted "sex all the time" like I'd heard about when I was growing up. Trouble is, I never found him. Oh well.

This woman was so consumed by the lack of affection and connection to her husband that she had lost sight of what prompted his drop in desire in the first place: losing a sibling can be devastating.

If your husband has experienced a loss recently, chances are his lack of desire is brought about by his suffering. Since grief has no universal timetable—that is, everyone grieves differently and for different lengths of time—grief has to run its course. If you think your husband needs professional help to assist him through his pain and may need addiitional motivation to seek help, he might benefit from the information on my Web site www.sexstarvedwife.com.

Elisabeth Kübler-Ross identified in her book, *On Death and Dying*, the five stages of grief:

Denial—the stage when people simply can't believe that what happened actually happened. They say to themselves, "There must be some mistake. This isn't really happening." In a sense, they are in a state of shock.

Anger—when people get angry at the person who died or God or blame themselves or others for what happened. "How could you die on me?" "How could this be happening to me? I don't deserve this."

Bargaining—the stage when people attempt to negotiate a different outcome. Although a different outcome is usually impossible, it doesn't stop them from replaying the "deals" over and over in their minds. For instance, someone who has been diagnosed with a serious illness such as lung cancer might be telling himself, "Just let me get over this, and I promise, I will *never* smoke cigarettes again."

Sadness or depression—the stage when people allow themselves to feel the despair that is often inevitable with loss. They often feel defeated, and life can lose meaning. People can even feel suicidal.

Acceptance—when people finally accept that life goes on regardless of the loss. It doesn't mean that you forget what happened or that you stop feeling sad, but the overwhelming feelings of grief fade. There is a recommitment to life and a refocus on the future.

No two people go through these stages exactly the same way or at the same time. In fact, not everyone goes through all the stages. But knowing that there are typical feelings people have as they move through the grieving process can help you better understand your husband.

JOB LOSS

Involuntary unemployment, especially for older men, can be nothing short of devastating because men's self-esteem is often so wrapped up in their professional identity. Recent research suggests that up to one in seven men who become unemployed will become depressed. Then, to make matters worse, depressed people have a hard time finding the motivation to do a serious job search, and if they manage to get themselves an interview, they often don't make a great impression because they feel down in the dumps. When they don't get the job, it's yet another rejection. Under these circumstances, the last thing on your husband's mind will be making love to you. He's in another world. His interest will return when he makes peace with what has happened and looks at his life circumstance as a new positive challenge or becomes employed again. Unless you have lots of contacts that might result in his finding new employment, the only thing you can do is to help him create a better, more productive outlook on what has happened in his life. Let's take a look at some ways you might do that.

Empathy

If your husband lost his job and is withdrawn, angry, irritable, or depressed, you can safely assume that he is truly suffering. He will in fact be going through the five stages of grieving mentioned above. Before you try to lift his spirits by telling him to look on the bright side of things, it is essential that he feels that you understand the depth of his feelings. See if you can identify in which stage he presently finds himself. Even if you think he's wallowing in his sadness, talk to him, let him talk to you, and show your caring and concern. Ask him what you can do to help him feel better. Tell him you understand; all people like to feel understood, especially when they're going through a hard time.

Help Him Set Goals

Your husband probably hasn't been in the mood to set goals for himself. If he's open to it, you could help him set solution-oriented goals. Veer away from overly ambitious goals such as, "I will be gainfully employed." Hopefully, that will happen, but you want to help him set smaller goals, goals he can accomplish quickly. For instance, "Tomorrow I will review three newspapers' classified sections and look at monster.com. Plus I will send out at least four résumés." Notice that these goals are short term and do not rely on any particular response from employers. They just require that your husband take some small action. These are the kinds of goals that, when accomplished, will help him feel as if he's making progress. And seeing that he's making progress is inspirational.

Offer Encouragement

Once your husband starts to take baby steps away from his funk, you should compliment him on his progress. Even if the steps are small, it helps for you to acknowledge them because he will have a hard time noticing good things that he's doing. People who are down feel down about themselves. You can lend another perspective.

And while I'm on the subject of encouragement, feel free to say and do nice things to him in regard to *anything* that you notice that merits praise. His ego needs building now.

Focus on His Strengths

Since his ego has been tied up in his being a provider for the family, it will be helpful for you to notice other ways in which he contributes to the family now that he is unemployed. Feeling dispensable is dispiriting. Make sure you do what you can to help him feel needed. For example, your husband may be more available for child care or housekeeping responsibilities. If this is true, let him know how much it means to you that your home life in humming due to his involvement.

Stop Doing More of the Same

I've worked with so many wives of unemployed men who, out of frustration, keep doing the same old thing over and over, with pretty miserable results. Here's an example.

Martha's husband, Luke, age fifty-six, had worked at the same company for seventeen years. He always believed he would retire there, but the company downsized, and management positions were the first to go. Luke's job was at the top of the list. It completely caught Luke by surprise.

Nevertheless, he was pleased with his severance package and thought that he'd be up and running with another job within a few months. But that new job didn't materialize.

Although their sex life had always been satisfying to both of them, now Luke was completely disinterested. When he stopped initiating sex, Martha took over and made sexual advances. But not only did Luke not want sex, he didn't want *any* sort of physical affection. Martha was distraught. She was apprehensive about their financial future. She also worried about Luke and felt distanced from him.

As time passed, Martha felt that it was important for her to help Luke because he seemed to be at a standstill. When Martha returned from her job each night, she would ask Luke about his day and about his job search efforts. At first, Luke filled her in with his day's activities. Martha found herself offering him many suggestions of things he could do differently the next day and in the days to come. Initially, Luke was receptive to her comments, but he eventually became annoyed that Martha was "hovering over him." Although she assured him that she was just trying to help, Luke thought otherwise. Martha thought that Luke was starting to feel sorry for himself and that he wasn't tackling things with a positive attitude. The more she tried to advise him on this matter, the more upset Luke got. The more upset Luke became, the more their marriage deteriorated. That's when Martha scheduled an appointment with me to see what could be done about her tense, financially strained, sexless marriage.

After talking with her, it became clear that Martha was doing several things that were unproductive. By now, I bet you can tell what they are. Luke felt that Martha had become an overbearing parent, constantly checking on him and offering suggestions that he experienced as criticisms. Furthermore, Martha realized that his unemployment had become the focus of their lives. Whatever happened to the children, friends, family, walks around the block, going to church together, or just simply spending quiet time together when they talked about anything other than his lack of work? Martha hadn't recognized how problem focused she had become. Furthermore, she had also been pressuring him regularly about his loss of interest in sex, which never resulted in his being more sexual.

When we discussed her more-of-the-same behaviors, Martha was quite eager to experiment with something different. She realized that, in her effort to help Luke, he was feeling undermined and usurped, not great for an already bruised male ego. We came up with a plan.

For the next two weeks, Martha agreed to avoid initiating any conversation about Luke's job search and to instead focus on more positive topics. She was to apologize to Luke for being so critical when she knew in her heart of hearts that he was going to handle things well and that things were going to turn out just fine. She agreed to resist the temptation to fine-tune Luke's ideas about finding work even if she thought she had a better plan. I suggested that when Luke shared information with her, she simply say, "That sounds great. Let me know what happens." Additionally, Martha realized that she had put aside many other areas of her life that were important to her, such as family members and church-related activities. I gave Martha "permission" to get her life back.

Martha followed through with all the homework tasks that we discussed. Luke seemed a bit surprised, to say the least, when she apologized. She could also tell that he was waiting for the third degree every night when she came home. However, after a few nights of her coming home and being pleasantly upbeat, she noticed Luke's mood changing as well. The more she accepted the situation, the more relaxed Luke became. The more relaxed and confident Luke became, the more energy he had to focus on the tough work of finding new employment. Martha saw that their relationship was moving in a positive direction, and that gave her hope. Some of the "old Luke" was returning. Although he had yet to find a full-time job, he had been offered a temporary part-time position. This was not his ultimate dream job, and Martha was concerned that by his taking it, he would stop looking for a better job. But as she promised, she resisted the temptation to guide him. Luke started laughing again, being more physically affectionate, and they even had sex twice by the end of my work with her. I could see they were moving in the right direction when we parted.

Back to you. Make sure you're clear about what you need to stop doing and stop doing it immediately. Once you stop doing what hasn't been working, commit to approaching your husband's period of unemployment with creativity. If you want more physical affection, your husband has to feel supported, connected, and appreciated because he's a little lost right now.

MIDLIFE CRISIS

Has your marriage been seemingly good until the day your husband woke up and looked around, only to discover that he is unhappy about practically everything in his life? He offers up a long list of the various aspects of his day-to-day existence that are meaningless, unsatisfying, and unrewarding. And oh, by the way, did you notice that you and everything you represent is way on top of the list? He loves you, but he's not in love with you anymore. He isn't affectionate and doesn't want to be close physically in any way. Welcome to your midlife crisis husband.

My husband had all the classic midlife crisis lines: "I'm not in love with you anymore, we've grown apart, we have nothing in common, we fight about everything, we are exact opposites, etc." He moved out for a while but moved back in again. We are doing a lot better communicating, but dreadful in the bedroom. We have talked about my sexual issues, and he says he can't just have sex with me; it has to be love, and he is not in love with me. He is just sitting back waiting for the "magical" feeling of love to spontaneously come back. I am at a loss as to what to do.

I had been up and down with my weight all my adult life. At this point, I was up. He told me he didn't desire me because of my weight. So I lost thirty pounds, and he still didn't want me. Then there was the excuse about our master bedroom, which was on the second floor. He said he didn't want to sleep up there because it was hot. I'm always cold; he's always hot. He moved downstairs and left the windows open all night. It was freezing down there, and I couldn't sleep, so I stayed upstairs.

In the meantime we haven't had sex for six months. The last time we did have sex, I could tell he was forcing himself to do it. It was physically satisfying but emotionally empty. I felt like a hooker, used, and like the most undesirable woman on the planet. I just want to feel connected to my husband. I want to feel loved and desired as a woman. I need physical touch to feel special. All the things he could do before but not now. Why???? Now all I get is the kiss goodbye in the morning and good night—the same way you would kiss a child. It makes me so sad.

Despite what your husband says, you are not the cause of all of his un-happiness. While there might be some things about your relationship that need improvement, his unhappiness has much more to do with is-sues that are going on for him personally. He just happens to be strik-ing out at you because you're within close range. However, knowing that you're not entirely to blame for his existential dilemma won't do a bit of good for your sex life. It may help you feel better about yourself, which is good, but you need more of a plan to get your sex life back on track.

Here are some do's and don'ts for dealing with a midlife crisis man.

• *Vanishing sex may just be the tip of the iceberg.*

If your husband has been rejecting your sexual advances or ignoring your pleas for more sexual intimacy and he's in the middle of a midlife cri-sis, your sex life isn't the only thing in trouble. Your marriage might be on the chopping block. When people are unhappy, they often falsely believe that leaving a situation will bring happiness. Despite the fact that you're lacking physical affection, you might have to put that need on the back burner for a while until your husband becomes a bit more certain that he's staying. In other words, now's not a good time to make a huge issue about your sexual relationship. Your complaints might be the excuse he needs to leave. But what should you do in the meantime?

• *Don't expect overnight miracles.*

Even if your husband gave you the "I love you, but I'm not in love with you" line just last night, his feelings didn't begin yesterday. His neg-ative thoughts have been percolating for quite a while. Generally a man mulls things over for months, even years, before he tells you how miser-able he really is, and it is precisely for that reason that you shouldn't ex-pect him to feel differently quickly. Recovering from a midlife crisis takes time; the length of time required varies from man to man. I don't want you to get your hopes up and think that things will improve instantly. They won't.

• *Listen and be a friend.*

Although it's highly possible that your husband won't want to talk much at all about his confusion with life right now, he might. And if he does, you should be his friend. Listen without judgment. If that's not possible, and it may not be, you can judge—but keep it to yourself. Let him know that you hear him and that it must be very confusing to feel those new feelings and that you have faith that he will make the right decisions about his life. If you can identify with any small part of what he's saying, let him know that.

If you start to worry that because you're not calling him on his erratic or irresponsible behavior, it might appear that you're condoning his actions, you're not. The only thing you're doing is avoiding confrontation, which will quickly polarize the two of you. You are avoiding burning bridges behind you or making matters worse. And when your husband eventually emerges out of his fog, he will think of you as his friend rather than an enemy. That's a good thing.

• *Be patient.*

It goes without saying that when you're desperate for physical affection, waiting a while feels like waiting an eternity. This means that you are going to have to be *very* patient. You will have to find ways to avoid being reactive to his distorted thinking. You will have to discover techniques for biting your tongue. In short, you are going to have to let this phase in your life and your marriage run its course.

You are going to have faith that if you sit back, sit tight, and let your husband do his thing for a while, he will eventually come to his senses and realize what a good thing he's got going with you. However, he has to arrive at this conclusion himself. I know this is a difficult thing to do, but in my years of working with women whose husbands had been abducted by the midlife crisis alien, the ones who were successful at rebuilding passion in their lives with their husbands were the ones who didn't overreact when their husbands left planet earth.

To help you do this, think about some other time in your life that you needed to be amazingly patient. Recall what was going on back then and how you recognized the importance of remaining calm and centered regardless of what was going on around you. What did you tell yourself that enabled you to take one day at a time? Or better yet, one minute at a time. Whatever resources you utilized in the past are still within you. You can access them again. I know you can.

Don't try to reason with or convince your husband that he isn't seeing things clearly: Although it might seem logical to tell him that he's just going through a phase that will pass, pull out the photo albums to reminisce about the good old days, or reassure him that all couples go through hard times and that you will get through this together, it will backfire. When he tells you that he loves you but he's not in love with you anymore, if you insist that his feelings will return, he won't buy it. In fact, the more you try to convince him, the more stubbornly he holds on to his pessimism about everything. What's worse, he feels that you just don't understand him, and it makes him even more withdrawn from you. As hard as it might be, you simply can't try to talk him out of his midlife crisis.

• Don't offer advice.

Here's the tricky part. Even if you possess the best advice in the world, your husband won't be receptive to it at the moment, because more than anything else, he wants to be the designer of his own life. He wants to call the shots. Any advice you offer will be flat-out rejected. That's just part of the midlife crisis syndrome. I know you are full of great suggestions, but it doesn't really matter what I think. What matters is what your husband thinks, and for right now, you know the drill—no advice.

• Don't ask questions or make demands.

What I'm about to say is unquestionably unfair, so steel yourself. Despite the fact that your husband may be withdrawn, edgy, insensitive, and self-centered, now's not the time to make demands of him. Don't give him ultimatums that his behavior has to change or you're leaving. Don't tell him that either he goes with you to counseling or he's out. Don't turn up the heat sexually and insist that he take your needs into account. If you do, he will, in all likelihood, leave. And I assume you don't want that to happen.

There's another thing you shouldn't do right now if your husband is truly in the throes of a midlife crisis: ask him a million questions about his plans, whereabouts, thoughts, and feelings. Although I believe you have a right to all of this information, if he feels cornered, trapped, or interrogated, he will resist.

• *Expect a roller coaster ride.*

Fasten your seat belt. There are many ups and downs in the lives of couples coping with a midlife crisis. Your husband's uncertainty about what he wants in life and how to accomplish that will create real inconsistencies in how he acts, feels, and responds and what he says to you. One day, all hell will be breaking loose, and the next, everything will seem okay. The alien who abducted your husband has returned him. One day he will behave with a great sense of entitlement, the next with remorse. As you go through this period, try hard not to take any of his moods, declarations, or actions to heart. Tomorrow they might be different.

• *Focus on yourself.*

With all these ups and downs, how in the world are you supposed to keep your sanity? Good question. You need to ask yourself, "If my husband fell off the face of the earth and I was single again, what would I need to do to make myself happy?" Be really specific with your answer, and then start doing those things. You need to keep focused on yourself and engage in activities that offer you strength, solace, and comfort. Here are some things women do while they're waiting out the storm.

> Focus on their children.
> Spend time with friends and family.
> Focus more on work.
> Get involved in religious or spiritual activities.
> Read.
> Start a new hobby.
> Do volunteer work.
> Keep a journal.
> Exercise regularly.

Here's one more thought to consider: get some therapy for yourself, or join a support group. It's important to have support, but it's essential that you seek out the kind of help that will be supportive of your marriage. Too many therapists or support groups take commitment to marriage too lightly. When problems occur, these therapists often declare the marriages dead on arrival. I know you don't want that for your marriage, or you wouldn't be so concerned about being close to your husband. So be careful about the choices you make when seeking help. Visit divorcebusting.com for marriage-friendly resources.

THERE IS HOPE

If your husband has pulled away from you sexually because nothing seems right in his life and he feels you're to blame, I know it's difficult for you right now. But I also know that there is hope. I have seen many couples survive midlife crises. And if you need a little inspiration, read this letter from a woman whose confused husband finally came home.

> Dear Michele,
>
> Last year at this time (Valentine's Day) I was an emotional wreck! My husband informed me, again, how miserable he was and how he needed to leave us (married seventeen years and three children). He told me he did not love me and never had loved me—That I was his problem and he wanted to find happiness and passion without me. I suspected an emotional affair with another woman. I remember so well waiting to see if I would get a card from my husband that had any words of affection. Of course, there wasn't! I shed many tears that day.
>
> However, here I am a year later, and my husband is "in love" with me again and can't stop telling me or showing me! Well, I am here to tell you that your methods work, and you CAN save your marriage BY YOURSELF, if you really want to put forth the time, effort and PATIENCE that it will take.
>
> MY suggestions:
>
> Don't push your husband into therapy with you! Men hate relationship talks, and if they resist therapy, go by yourself!

Don't insist on talks about your relationship.

Don't pry and become obsessed with other women he might be seeing.

Work on yourself!

Actions speak louder than words. Change *your* behavior and attitudes now! The only person you have any control over in this world is you!!!!

Don't pursue your husband . . . lovingly distance!

I am so happy with my husband's "recovery" and our wonderful NEW marriage. I feel like I am on my honeymoon again after seventeen years. I have no anger or unresolved feelings now that my husband is surrounding me with such love. I have grown so much over the past year and have much success in many areas to show for it. You see, I was unhappy too, just in denial over the dismal shape of my marriage. I don't appreciate the way that my husband rocked my world, but I am better for it in many ways.

CHAPTER NINE

Working It Out Together

The Secret to a Long Marriage

With a couple celebrating their fiftieth anniversary at the church's marriage marathon, the minister asked Brother Ralph to take a few minutes and share some insight into how he had managed to live with the same woman all these years.

The husband replied to the audience, "Well, I treated her with respect, spent money on her, but mostly I took her traveling on special occasions."

The minister inquired, "Trips to where?"

"For our twenty-fifth anniversary, I took her to Beijing, China."

The minister then said, "What a terrific example you are to all husbands. Ralph, please tell the audience what you're going to do for your wife on your fiftieth anniversary?"

Ralph replied, "I'm going to go get her."

I think it's pretty safe to say that when there is a desire gap in marriage, there are relationship issues that need work. This doesn't mean that all desire gap problems are *caused* by marital problems. It's often the other way around: many marital problems are the *result* of a sexual desire gap.

It's also safe for me to assume that although this chapter is about relationship solutions, you are the one in charge of making sure many of these solutions happen. I want to reassure you that that is okay. In fact, it's more than okay. Relationships are such that if one person changes, the relationship changes. So you don't have to try to strong-arm your husband to read this chapter with you. You can get the ball of change rolling all by yourself. I say, "It takes one to tango."

If you're skeptical, let me give you an example that will change your mind. Let's imagine that you are having a great evening with someone you love. You are having a wonderful conversation, and good feelings are flowing. It's an evening to be remembered. And then for some reason, you decide that you want the evening to go downhill. Can you think of something that you could say or do that would turn the evening sour? I bet as you're reading this, you're smiling. Of course, you can.

When I ask this question in my couples' seminars, someone always responds, "I could definitely ruin the evening if I wanted to. I know exactly how to push his buttons." Sound familiar? If you know how to push your husband's buttons in a negative way, you can learn how to push your husband's buttons in a positive way. Everyone has within him positive change buttons. You just have to know how to find and activate them, and I will help you do that.

Some of the solutions are designed simply to help you and your spouse get along better. The theory is that once you work out your differences, he will want to feel closer sexually. Other sexual stalemates have more to do with sexual issues in particular, and you will find solutions to these sorts of problems as well. As usual, read through all the solutions, and see what makes sense to you. Experiment, watch the results, and keep doing it if it's working. Try something else if it's not.

THE CATCH-22

Conventional wisdom suggests that gender differences account for out-of-sync sexuality between men and women. It is said that women need to feel close and connected to their partners emotionally before they're interested in being sexual. Men, they say, need to feel close and connected physically before they invest themselves emotionally. Women wait for their husbands to spend time and romance them and have intimate conversations before they want to have sex. Men wait for their wives to flirt, touch, hold, and kiss them, or initiate sex before they're interested in spending time together, going out on dates, or having tête-à-têtes.

But I'm here to tell you that in many relationships, it is just the opposite—*men* need to feel in sync emotionally in order to desire their wives, while women need touch in order to feel emotionally connected to their husbands. You know this better than anyone.

Brent, a client of mine some years ago, taught me a thing or two about relationships and sexuality. He was in his mid-forties at the time and a high-powered attorney. Brent had various complaints about his marriage, and one of them was a lackluster sex life. He and his wife rarely made love. As I heard him tell his story, I began to formulate stereotypical and erroneous ideas about what was happening in his marriage. I asked him, "Isn't she interested in making love?" His answer caught me off guard: "That's not it," he replied. "*I'm* the one who isn't interested." I asked him why, and he told me that his wife was highly critical. From his perspective, she was always complaining about the marriage, telling him what he was doing wrong, not appreciating any of his contributions to the family—his financial support, his care for the children—and finding fault with him no matter how hard he tried. And then he said, "I have absolutely no interest in being close to her physically when she is critical or picks on me. I don't want to get near her at all. All she ever does is hurt my feelings."

At that point in my career, I had heard those thoughts expressed only by women. I wasn't accustomed to hearing men turn down sex because of hurt feelings. But in the intervening years, I have heard from countless men who feel exactly the same way that Brent did. When their wives are critical, angry, demeaning, short, or moody, the last thing they feel like doing is being close physically. You probably have lots of friends who tell you that their husbands want sex no matter what is happening in the marriage, but for millions of men, it just ain't so. And perhaps you're married to one of them. If you are, the first thing you need to do is to make sure your irritability, anger, or critical nature isn't pushing your spouse away. Feelings of hurt, anger, resentment, and disappointment may be what are standing in the way of his wanting to reach out to you. If so, you will need to work on the foundation of your marriage in order to spark his sexual interest.

Start with thinking about the following questions:

- If I were talking to your husband and you were out of the room, would he say that you are more complimentary or critical?
- Does he often tell you to get off his back and stop criticizing him?
- Do you frequently find yourself focusing on the things he does wrong?
- Are you almost always angry toward him?

As you think about these questions, I want you to be honest with yourself.

Do you think you've been harsher with your spouse than in times past when things were better between you? If you have, I completely understand why you've been irritable with him; you've been unhappy, you've been hurt, you've been feeling rejected. I suspect that if your husband were to make mad love to you, you would definitely be less critical. You would want to lavish him with praise. Hopefully, he will eventually come toward you and be more affectionate. But in the meantime, you've really got to work hard at bolstering the emotional closeness in your marriage if you want your husband to come closer to you. I know that it's hard for you to think about being kind, loving, complimentary, and appreciative when you feel cheated or denied. I never told you that this was going to be easy, but you have to do it anyway. What's the "it" you have to do? Start by applying many of the relationship-building strategies in this chapter. Notice that the first homework tasks are things you do outside your bedroom, and none of them includes talking about sex. That comes later.

SPEAK HIS LOVE LANGUAGE

One book I like very much is *Five Love Languages*, by Gary Chapman. Chapman explains that we all have different ways of feeling loved, and each person has his or her own "love language." In good marriages, people work very hard at speaking their partner's love language even if they don't quite understand or identify with it. If you want your husband to feel closer to you, you have to speak his language. Chapman believes that people feel loved:

- When their partner spends quality time with them
- Through encouraging words and conversations
- When they receive gifts from their spouse
- Through acts of service—when their spouse does things to please them, such as cleaning the house, warming a car before traveling on a cold wintry evening, taking the clothes to the cleaners, and so on
- Through physical touch

As you read these five languages of love, perhaps you were thinking about your own love languages. Do you think maybe physical touch is one of them? You don't have to limit it to only one; you might have a blend of two or more love languages. Now think about your husband's love language. If it's not touch, what is it? His turn-on is probably something you do outside the bedroom. Identify *his* turn-on, and think about what you can do for him. Here's an example.

Chrissie and Wes were married for five years and had no children. Chrissie was an extremely physical person who described herself as "touchy-feely." Her parents were very loving and physically affectionate people, and that's where she learned about the importance of touch. To Chrissie, touch meant love. Chrissie was unhappy with the frequency with which she and Wes made love. She also wanted Wes to spend more time touching, cuddling, or just holding hands.

Wes had his own set of disappointments in their marriage. Although his parents weren't physical, they had other ways of showing their love. In particular, his mother was a dedicated stay-at-home mom and fabulous cook. She was the sort who volunteered at school, sponsored big bake sales, and made wonderful dinners for the family.

Although Chrissie loved Wes very much, she was quite driven professionally and had big career ambitions. She was not particularly interested in home-cooked meals and had no other Martha Stewart–like inclinations. When Wes complained about her lack of interest in their home or in taking part in mealtime preparations, Chrissie would get infuriated by what she thought of his "small-minded" requests. Wes felt that she valued her career over him. The more they fought about their lifestyle choices, the less sex they had.

When I met with Chrissie, I talked to her about their love languages. I convinced her to look at Wes's requests for home-cooked meals through different lenses. I suggested that she go home and begin to do some of the family-oriented things for which Wes had been yearning. I told her to stop putting him down for wanting those things and to be more invested in real giving.

At first, she was a bit resistant because she had been feeling so hurt by Wes's "coldness," and she had also thought that Wes's requests were "sexist." She asked a question that many women ask when I give them a homework assignment: "Why do *I* have to be the one to change?" "That's a good question," I told her. "You don't have to 'be the one to change;' you merely need to tip over the first domino. And when you do and Wes starts coming closer to you, the only question you'll ask yourself is, 'Why did I wait so long?' "

Despite all of her reservations, Chrissie decided to start putting more energy into pleasing Wes in his way. She cooked more for him and tried to create a warmer, cozier, more comfortable feeling in their home. The more she softened toward him, the more he lightened up in her presence. He seemed happier, they talked more, they spent more time together, and he definitely became more physical. Although Chrissie still hoped for more frequent sex, she agreed that their sex life had definitely improved.

PAY ATTENTION TO HIS STRENGTHS

If your husband is harboring feelings of resentment, hurt, or anger and feeling disconnected from you, he will be particularly sensitive to anything you say or do that feels to him like a put-down. The best remedy is for you to do your absolute best to notice and comment on anything he does or says that is positive. I know this is difficult when you're feeling vulnerable because of his rejection, but you need to be the one to tip over the domino.

Here's your assignment. In the days ahead, I want you to make a point of complimenting your husband at least two or three times a day. Let him know how much you appreciate something he's done or that he's good at. If you notice that he's trying to be cooperative with you in any way, acknowledge it out loud. (I have many women in my practice who tell me that they notice some of the good things their husbands do and consider saying something about it but then forget.) I once had a woman in my practice tell her husband, "I know what just happened would have typically pissed you off, but you didn't get angry, so I'm impressed." In other words, the absence of annoying behavior is worthy of comment as well. See if your more positive focus triggers a positive change in him. It may happen immediately, or it may take a few days or weeks. Look for the small signs that he's feeling closer to you. He may hang out with you more. He may initiate conversation more readily. He may call from work just to say hello. He may be willing to do more around the house or with the kids. He may compliment you in return. And he may (drum roll please!) become more physically affectionate. You may even want to keep a journal of the positive things you say and his reactions. This will help you become clearer about strategies that work. You will also feel encouraged by the "proof" of your progress!

CHOOSE YOUR BATTLES WISELY

The worst possible advice you could give to a newlywed couple is, "Express your feelings openly and honestly all the time." That is truly a formula for disaster. If you talk to couples who have been married for a long time and have a sound relationship, they will laugh at the idea of free-for-all honesty. People are a package deal; you will have some things you love about them and some things that you really don't like at all. In good relationships, you have to learn how to let the small things slide. You can't be calling your spouse on every little thing that irritates you; you'd be fighting all the time. This is especially true if your husband is allergic to conflict.

So here's the deal: if and when you start to feel annoyed, irritated, or upset with your husband's behavior, ask yourself, "Is what I'm about to say or do going to help us feel closer and more connected or push us further away?" If your goal is to build on positive feelings, restrain yourself. I am in no way saying that you should keep all of your feelings to yourself and just stew about them. If something is really important to you, then by all means discuss it. But first wait fifteen minutes, cool down, and then reevaluate whether it's still something worth discussing.

When you hit on something that needs to be addressed, it's essential to have a collaborative conversation. Reread Chapter 6 to refresh yourself about the best ways to approach heated topics.

APPROACH THE CONFLICT AVOIDER

As you were reading the previous suggestions, you might be thinking, "This doesn't apply to us because we never fight!" Some of the most challenging types of relationships I've encountered are the ones where one spouse keeps all negative thoughts and feelings to himself or herself. Well, I shouldn't say *all*, because eventually one small, seemingly insignificant thing happens, and it becomes the straw that breaks the camel's back. But because the reaction is so dramatic given the size of the infraction, the outcry gets labeled as "overreaction," or "unreasonable," and is flatly ignored. Then months or even years can go by without so much as a word when things go awry. This is, without question, an excellent way to avoid conflict. It's also the best way to kill feelings of intimacy and desire.

Is your husband someone who hates conflict and refuses to rock the boat? Do you sometimes sense that he's angry at you but says nothing? Guys like your husband who will do just about anything to avoid an argument end up shutting down emotionally and physically. Does this sound familiar?

If you think that your husband may be a conflict avoider, that may be what is dampening his feelings for you. You need to give him the opportunity to share what's on his mind. In fact, you need to insist. Sit him down—at a time when things are quiet and you can talk without being interrupted—and tell him that you know he's unhappy about something and you need to know what's going on with him. Let him know that you're aware that you're not perfect, and neither is your marriage, but you're open to hearing his feelings about anything you could do differently. Help him feel safe to share what's going on with him without fear of your defending yourself or attacking in return.

If he stalls, don't let him off the hook. He might squirm, wiggle, get upset, sigh deeply, or even seem annoyed, but just keep showing your interest in knowing more about his feelings. I worked with a couple who, when the woman asked her husband to talk about sex, the husband cried. She couldn't stand his tears so she avoiding talking about sex; he had trained her to steer clear of a very important subject. I, on the other hand, didn't allow his tears to halt our talk about sex. I just handed him the tissues.

If your husband still avoids you, write him a letter. Send him an e-mail. Call him on his cell phone. Just make sure you give him ample opportunity to open up. Even if what he has to say is less than pleasant, it's been my experience that once things are out in the open, there is potential for healing and connection.

One word of caution: if you know you are married to a conflict avoider and your question, "Honey, what's wrong?" prompts silence or anger in him, this particular approach isn't for you. Always remember that insanity has been defined as doing the same old thing and expecting different results.

What if you're *both* reluctant to talk about what's bothering you? I worked with a couple where both spouses were conflict avoiders. Whenever either partner was unhappy about something, both avoided it like the plague. From the outside, everyone thought they had the perfect marriage. They were financially successful, physically attractive, had lots of close relationships with family and friends. But ten years into their marriage, the wife realized that the passion was gone. Sex was infrequent, and her attraction to her husband had faded. They were a perfect example of what happens in marriage when conflict avoidance becomes the top priority. Once I convinced them both to become more genuine with each other, the connection between them slowly returned.

If you are like your husband in your desire to keep things calm at home at all costs, you must face your fear of conflict and lead the way for the two of you. Research tells us that what separates people in long-term, happy marriages from those who divorce is their ability to handle conflict in a healthful way.

Throughout this book, I've emphasized the importance of having a vehicle for working out your differences. I'm not just talking about your sexual differences. I'm also talking about how you deal with your children, extended families, money, household chores, and choices about how free time is spent. If you feel that conversations about these tough subjects end up as shouting matches where things never get resolved, or uncomfortable debates leaving both of you in silence, or where one of you wants closure but the other has shut down, that's not a good thing. All couples need to feel that when something goes wrong, they have a method for fixing it. You need to trust that you can discuss important issues together, that you will listen to each other and take each other's feelings to heart. If you don't have this structure in your marriage, it can't feel safe. Without safety, you can't have real intimacy.

SEXY SOLUTIONS

The following "homework tasks" relate specifically to how you handle the "I'm hot, he's not" dynamic in your marriage. As with all the other solutions I've discussed, some will fit for you, while others might not. Start with the ones that appeal to you. They have been field-tested and proven helpful to many, many couples. See which ones work for you.

Focus on the Exceptions (Again)

No matter what kind of problem you're experiencing or how long it has been going on, there are undoubtedly times when things have been considerably better. However, it is human nature to focus on and emphasize things going wrong. Knowing how we tend to focus on difficulties and overlook the good times, I always ask about exceptions. I say, "I know things have been tough, but what's different about the times the two of you are getting along better? What are each of you doing differently?" People are typically stymied. They simply haven't been paying much attention to problem-free times, or if they notice them, they assume the good times are flukes. People assume good times just happen. Bad times, on the other hand, are caused by their partners.

The good times don't just happen. When things are going better, it's because each partner is doing something different. Here's an example.

Belinda and her husband, Paul, are both fifty-five years old. Paul had seemed to have sex on his mind day and night for many years of their marriage. But when I first met Belinda, Paul wanted sex only every other week, though he would concede to once a week if pressured.

That was not acceptable to Belinda, who wanted sex two or three times a week. What she missed most about their sexual relationship, however, was Paul's passion. She told me, "It is a wonderful feeling to have your husband want you the way he does when he is full of passion. The way he watches you . . . touches you . . . even kind of 'sucks up to you' when he wants sex. It's all part of the mating game, and I really miss that." Belinda felt that Paul basically adopted the philosophy, "If we do it, fine. If we don't, fine. It's not important to me anymore."

Rather than focus on what *was* working in their sexual relationship, Belinda immersed herself in what wasn't happening and all the bad feelings that went along with that. She felt sad and resentful much of the time and was not able to hide her disappointments.

I asked Belinda, "Although I know things aren't the way you'd like them to be, what does Paul do right sexually? Even if his positive behavior happens infrequently or is just a baby step, what's different about times that go right?"

Belinda replied, "Paul has told me that he really is willing to try something to increase his desire. I know that many men aren't willing to do that. That's good, I guess." I asked her whether she ever told him that she appreciated his willingness to try something and she said, "No." I suggested she start by doing that.

Belinda was quiet for a moment, then said, "The other good news is that when he does decide to have sex, he has no trouble getting an erection. It's strong and hard!" Again, I wondered how often she told him how much she enjoyed his penis and how satisfied she felt when they had sex. Not surprisingly, although she told him that she had a good orgasm from time to time, she really didn't emphasize what a good lover he is. I suggested that she go home and make a big deal about his being quite the Don Juan. Belinda followed through with my suggestion, with good results. Although the frequency of their lovemaking hadn't changed (yet), Paul was more passionate and caring about her feelings during sex.

Zoe also improved her sexual relationship with her husband, Jeff, by focusing on exceptions. Jeff seemed increasingly less interested in sex, which troubled her greatly. When I asked her what was different about times when he seemed more interested, she told me, "Before we had kids, Jeff was much more interested." I asked her what was different between them before the kids were born. Zoe told me that sex was more spontaneous. Now, with the kids always around, they had to have planned sex dates, and that was a turn-off for her husband. Then she said, "The only other thing I can think of is that in the past, I said dirty things when we screwed. I sent him e-mails with erotic messages. I stopped doing that because I've been mad about his lack of interest in me sexually. I hadn't thought about that until you asked the question, but now that I think about it, he really used to get fired up when I talked dirty."

It became clear that by doing two things, Zoe would improve her chances that Jeff would be more turned on. First, she needed to think of ways to introduce spontaneity and creativity into their lovemaking. Without telling Jeff, she got her kids invited for sleepovers at friends' houses. When he came home, she seduced him with sexy lingerie and a sexy video. It worked like a charm.

Zoe also employed her sure-fire passion-building technique of the past—talking dirty—and realized quickly that the old trick still worked. Once Zoe reapplied those techniques to her marriage, she discovered that some things never change. And for her, that was a good thing.

Now let's get back to you. The following questions will help you identify exceptions that can turn into solutions. Think of a time in your marriage when your sexual relationship was better and ask yourself:

- What was my husband doing differently then?
- What was I doing differently back then?
- How was I treating my spouse differently?
- What was different about my life during that time?
- What was different about our lives together?
- What was different about our family?

When you focus on exceptions to the problem, you'll be focusing on solutions. And as Martha Stewart would say, "That's a good thing."

Stop Doing More of the Same

Sometimes the very thing you do to resolve a problem becomes the problem. Let me explain.

When there's a problem in life, people generally do something to fix it. If the solution works, all's right in the world. If what we do doesn't work, instead of saying to ourselves, "That didn't work—time to do something entirely different," we usually tell ourselves, "That didn't work; guess I didn't say it loudly enough or do it with enough determination. I'll need to do it one more time, this time with feeling." You know what I mean? And guess what happens when you do more of what hasn't been working? If you're thinking, "Things stay the same," you're wrong. Things do not stay the same; they get worse.

Think about parents who discover that they have a sneaky teenager. What do they do? They begin to spy on their kid. But what happens when the kid discovers that his parents are spying? He gets sneakier, and the very behavior the parents were trying to eliminate has now gotten worse. Unfortunately the parents don't turn to one another and say, "Honey, that didn't work. Let's try a completely different approach," they say, "That kid! We really aren't on top of things! We'll have to spend more time and energy watching him closely and snooping in his things to make sure we know what's going on." And that sends the boy even further underground.

There is one more thing you should know about the "more-of-the-same" dilemma. Generally when people choose their approach to a problem, it is typically the most logical, straightforward thing to do. Spying on a sneaky person makes sense; the only problem is that it doesn't always work. In other words, just because your approach makes sense and is perfectly reasonable doesn't make it effective.

How does this apply to you? Let's say that when you started to notice that your husband was withdrawing sexually, my guess is you did what any logical woman would do—you talked to him about it. Perhaps he was even receptive to your discussion at first. However, when his receptivity didn't translate into his becoming more amorous, you probably concluded that it was time for talk again. This time you noticed that he seemed less patient and not nearly as receptive. In fact, he seemed rather annoyed. What was supposed to be a heart-to-heart talk ended up as an argument, with both of you going separate ways—hardly the response you were hoping for.

Time passes, nothing changes, and you assume it's time for talk number three. This time it results in an all-out argument with lots of nasty accusations and a subsequent two-week cold war. Think about it. You want more closeness and what you're getting is more distance. The harder you try to fix things, the worse things seem to get. Clearly it's time for a change.

The first thing you need to do is to figure out what you're doing—that is, more of the same. How can you tell when you're doing it? It's simple: you hit the same dead ends over and over. In fact, I bet there are certain things you've said or done repeatedly, and while you're in the midst of doing those things, you know full well what the outcome will be. And here's something else you need to know: although there are exceptions to every rule, many men tend to be less verbally oriented than women. If you happen to be married to a man of few words, no matter what you say or how you're saying it, you may be doing more of the same.

Men who are less verbally oriented are more likely to be action oriented. They don't get together with their male buddies to talk about their feelings; they do something action oriented, such as playing golf, going to a football game, or spending a few days together fishing. I've never been on one of those fishing trips, but I have a strong feeling that not much beyond "Pass the beer" is said. Yet if you ask these guys about their connection to their buddies, they will truly feel close. It's that male bonding thing.

Too many women talk and talk and talk in the hope that someday their words will get through to these guys. Have you ever said to yourself, "If I've said it once, I've said it a million times," or "It's in one ear and out the other," or "I talk until I'm blue in the face"? Have you and your husband had a particular discussion so many times that you know precisely what both of you will say? Do you know the script so well that if he got sick, could you be the understudy? If so, it's time for a change. Start by reducing your words, and take action. Which action you choose will depend on your situation and your husband's prior responses. But just quit gabbing; he's heard all he's going to hear.

Catherine felt completely ignored by her husband, Milt. He worked long hours, came home, ate dinner, watched television, and fell asleep on the couch, night after night after night. Catherine felt neglected emotionally, sexually, and spiritually. For years, she talked to Milt about her feelings, but nothing ever changed. He dozed by the television as she fumed around the house. She tried begging him to go to counseling, reading self-help books, yelling at him, and threatening him with divorce. Still, no changes.

Eventually Catherine had enough. She decided that rather than divorce Milt, she was going to get a life of her own. She was going to do whatever she had to do (short of infidelity) to feel happier and more satisfied. And so she did. She re-established her relationships with her women friends, started taking two new classes in the evening, rarely was home in time to make dinner for Milt, and made herself less available to him when he called from work. In other words, she drastically changed her actions.

It took about three weeks before Milt started to do a turnabout. He began to grill her about her whereabouts, express disappointment (and annoyance) that she was never at home anymore, and was decidedly more attentive to her when she was at home. All of this surprised Catherine. She hadn't changed her behavior to change Milt; she had simply reached her limit with his self-centered lifestyle. But she learned what so many other women in her shoes learn: when it comes to men, it's often easier done than said.

Now I want you to try to think about what your more-of-the-same behaviors are right now. Here are some questions that might help you diagnose your go-nowhere strategies. Write down your responses to the questions in a journal or notebook or on a separate piece of paper.

- Think of a troublesome situation or argument that arises on a regular basis. What is it about? If you can think of more than one, write that down too.
- What is your usual way of handling it? What do you say? What do you do?
- What's your partner's usual way of handling or responding to it? What does he say and do?
- When he stubbornly makes his point or acts a certain way, how do you typically respond?

If you are having any difficulty answering these questions, try the following one:

- Although you may not agree with your husband about this, what would he say *you* do that drives him nuts in regard to this problem? Don't be defensive; just answer the question.

Once you recognize your more-of-the-same behavior, you're more than halfway home. Start by making a promise to yourself that you will abandon your more-of-the-same strategy immediately. You can replace it with any number of approaches listed in this chapter.

Do Something Different

Have this be your mantra: *If what I'm doing isn't working, I need to do something different.* For example, if it seems as if you're about to get into a heated discussion or engage in an unpleasant and unproductive battle, stop for a moment and ask yourself, "What is my goal here? What do I really want to have happen? Is what I'm about to do going to move me closer to my goal or push me further away? And if the answer is, "Move me further away," don't do it. Do something different instead. Anything different has a better chance of working than doing the same old thing.

In relationships, we are often on automatic pilot. Our interactions are so routine that we barely have to think about what we do or say. When, out of the blue, something entirely different occurs, it gets our attention. We must respond in a new way. Let me give you an example.

Brenda and Ed, a two-career couple with busy schedules, generally had sex on weekends. This schedule worked out fine for both of them, except that they began to have disagreements about money that started every Friday night when they returned home from work. Because their weekend began with an argument, the rest of the weekend was miserable and sexless. This had been going on for two months. Brenda was very upset about the arguments and even more disturbed about the lack of intimacy in their marriage. She tried to talk to Ed about the unhealthy new pattern in their relationship, but when Fridays rolled around, like clockwork, a battle would inevitably break out. Brenda was determined to take a look at her role in the fights and see if there was something that she could do to bring about a more peaceful ending that would set the tone for physical close-ness later in the weekend. She came up with a plan.

The next Friday night, Ed initiated the usual conversation about money. Brenda listened patiently to his points and instead of disagreeing vehemently—her usual tactic—she said, "I want to talk to you about this. I really hear your point [and she reiterated his point], but I'm a little tired and would prefer waiting until Sunday to discuss this. Is that okay with you?" Surprised by her different response, Ed simply responded, "Okay, whatever."

Ed and Brenda decided to go out for dinner together and had a really good time. On Saturday, they decided to go to a movie and again had an enjoyable time together. Because things were clicking, Brenda decided to make a move sexually, and Ed responded positively. It was the first time in over two months that they had made love. By Sunday, they were feel-ing better about each other than they had for a long time, which proba-bly explains why, when Brenda brought up the money issue on Sunday night, they were able to resolve their differences. A simple change in Brenda's behavior changed the pattern between them that had kept them apart.

Figuring out what to do differently isn't as difficult as you might sus-pect. Just remind yourself of your more-of-the-same behavior and prom-ise yourself that you are going to do something different, no matter how weird or crazy it might seem at the time. You might not be as fortunate as Brenda and see the results instantaneously; you might have to wait a day or two, or more. Be patient, keep your eyes open, and look for small signs of change.

The Seesaw Effect

I mentioned the seesaw effect earlier in the book, but it bears repeating: the more you do something, the less your husband will do, and the more your husband does of something, the less you will do. This principle applies to all areas of relationships. For example, if you're always the one to send out birthday and holiday cards, your husband will count on your doing it and never think of doing it himself. If your husband handles every aspect of fi-nances in your family, chances are that you rarely think about the han-dling of money. If you are the emotional one in your relationship, it's likely that your husband keeps his emotions to himself. We tend to counterbalance one another. It's just human nature.

Have you ever had the experience of having a conversation with your husband, and although you don't exactly see eye to eye, you're not at opposite ends of the spectrum either? You're both talking about different shades of gray. But as the conversation continues, something shifts: you're saying, "Black," and he's saying, "White." That's because our positions are very fluid and we tend to react to each other strongly. We seesaw.

Let's take this analogy a step further. In many relationships, couples start out on equal footing when it comes to sexual desire. Then one person becomes tired, overwhelmed, preoccupied, or busy or has headaches. This new behavior prompts his or her spouse to double up efforts to keep their sex life on track. When their efforts are met with rejection, all of a sudden sex becomes the center of the universe for the sex-starved spouse. The more the sex-starved spouse shines a light on sex, the less sex the lower desire spouse wants.

> I have been married for only nine months. The only times my husband will have sex with me are on holidays and vacations. I am a complete mess. I realized this about our relationship about two months into marriage—he is a great person, and I care about him a lot, but he just doesn't need to have sex or have anything to do with sexual things, even kissing or hugs. We have no connection now—we have a brother-and-sister relationship. I can't stop obsessing. I am depressed and can't seem to want to do anything but sit in my house and not leave until he starts showing me that he wants me as a lover, not just as a partner.

The other interesting phenomenon is that spouses often take turns being the high-desire spouse and the low-desire spouse. In a sense, they play cat and mouse. Here's a letter from a guy who used to be the high-desire spouse but is no longer interested:

> I really like sex, so why don't I initiate it anymore? I fear rejection. It used to be that she liked sex all the time. Sex was her cure for things like headaches, etc. We always laughed at the shows where a

headache was the excuse; for her it was a reason to jump in bed. Then came the time where sex no longer worked like aspirin. She started to avoid sex, offering quite a variety of reasons. My available foreplay arsenal was no longer sufficient. So I quit trying. Now she's upset with me, and she wonders why I don't initiate or I'm not interested.

Suffice it to say that if you're the one putting all the energy into rekindling your sexual relationship, your husband has come to expect that. He knows you'll take the lead. It's time to make a change. If you want him to be more involved sexually, you need to experiment with stepping back and giving him a turn to notice you're not pursuing him.

When I make this suggestion to people, they often tell me that they've tried that without success. However, when I ask them how long they've backed off, it wasn't very long. After a few days or a few weeks, they could no longer contain themselves and either initiated sex once again or at least complained again about not having sex. If you don't wait long enough for your behavior to be noticed, you might as well not even do it. You have to be patient.

The other mistake women make when backing off is that they are silently stewing while they're doing it. In other words, they're so angry that they have to go to such great lengths to get their husbands to perk up that they storm around the house. But their husbands can tell there's a problem and they swiftly figure out what it might be. The goal is to act as if you've put sex on the back burner, and for the time being, you're truly not interested. This might kick your husband out of automatic pilot and pique his curiosity and, hopefully, his sex drive. This seesaw technique gives him a chance to pursue you without his feeling as if you coerced him.

Annie and her husband, Bill, behaved in a highly predictable pattern that lasted for several years. Annie would approach Bill for sex, he would decline, she would get angry, and then a couple of days later, he would approach her sexually. The problem was that Annie felt that his initiating sex was always out of a sense of obligation and that when they did make love, his heart really wasn't in it. Their lovemaking often left her feeling empty. Yet because Annie believed that the "I approach him—he rejects me—I get angry—he approaches me—we have sex" pattern was the only way they would end up being sexual, she continued to do what she always had done, even though sex was never truly satisfying.

After learning about the seesaw effect, Annie decided to try something new. As usual, she initiated sex with Bill, and he declined. As she predicted, two days passed. Then as he sat next to her on the couch, he began to rub her thighs. Instead of responding sexually this time (although she very much wanted to), she told him that she was really not in the mood. Thinking she was joking, Bill continued to touch her sexually. Eventually Annie asked him to stop and said, "I'm really not into this right now. I don't know why, but maybe some other time." Bill stopped and appeared somewhat stunned. He asked her if everything was okay, and she said, "Yes, absolutely. I'm just not feeling too sexual right now."

Bill clearly thought about Annie's response because when he was at work the next day, he sent her an e-mail with sexual undertones—something he had done early in their marriage but not for many years. Annie was tempted to respond in kind but held back. Later that evening, Bill made another sexual advance, kissing her in the kitchen and rubbing her butt. Annie kissed him but pulled away to finish the cleaning she had started. Again, this surprised Bill, who expected Annie to be ready to roll any time he showed interest.

After turning down a few more of Bill's sexual advances, Annie finally "gave in," and they made love. Apparently the wait did a world of good in terms of boosting Bill's enthusiasm for sex. "He seemed much more into it," Annie said. Rather than simply going through the motions, she felt connected and very turned on because of his improved passion.

Annie wasn't quite sure why her holding back made a difference to Bill, but it did. It wasn't easy for her to do; she worried that by resisting him, he would become even more low key sexually, but just the opposite happened.

Like Annie you too might worry that a new approach might backfire. That sort of concern is par for the course. It's scary to break free of old patterns, but you really have nothing to lose and everything to gain. So put your fears aside and give yourself permission to be creative.

Sex Talk Phobia

Although sex is everywhere—on television and radio, in magazines and newspapers—it's amazing how scary it is for couples to discuss their own sexual relationship. I've worked with many couples who panic when they sense that we're going to talk about sex. Too many people go for years feeling unhappy sexually but never really tell their partners about their feelings. They don't talk about what they enjoy or what turns them off. If they want more stimulation, faster or slower movements, different positions, more foreplay, less talking, more eye contact, they keep it a secret. They don't coach their spouses as to the best techniques for hitting home runs. Some people don't even make noise when they're feeling highly aroused.

One husband I worked with didn't want sex very often, and he told me that he hated the way his wife's breath smelled like cigarettes. I asked him if he had ever told her that, and he said, "No, I don't want to hurt her feelings." Which do you think hurts more: being rejected time and time again or hearing that your breath stinks and that perhaps you should brush your teeth or, better yet, quit smoking?

Another reason couples don't discuss their sex life is that they believe sex just happens; it's a "natural" act, and people should just know what to do. While it's true that any old sex can just happen, *good* sex doesn't just happen. Since no two people are alike, what turns each person on differs. If you want to be a good lover and have a hot sexual relationship, you've got to talk to each other. Leave mind-reading to the fortune-tellers.

Not talking about sex may be one reason that your sexual relationship isn't what it could be. If you are missing the mark in some way and you and your husband aren't discussing it, you won't know what you're doing "wrong." He might just be avoiding sex because something is missing, but he is keeping it to himself. Or he might have fears or reservations about sex that he's not sharing. They may be things you could help him with if only you knew what they were. Granted, talking about sex can be uncomfortable, especially if you're not used to it. But it's absolutely necessary, especially when things aren't going well.

Have you told your husband how you feel about your sexual relationship? Have you had specific talks about what your husband likes or dislikes about sex? Have you asked him what you can do differently that he might find more exciting? Many men tell me that they lose interest in sex because it becomes boring, routine, and unimaginative. They don't bother telling their wives about their feelings; they simply avoid sex.

But before you ask him about *his* feelings, you need to make sure that your husband knows how you've been feeling about your sexual relationship. I assume that you have already told him, but I am always surprised by the number of women who haven't been honest. Or if they have shared their feelings, it's been in anger, when their husbands have said no to sex. I want to quickly cover the obvious before moving on to other sex-enhancing ideas.

You need to tell your husband what you've been thinking and feeling about the distance between you sexually. Talk from your heart. Use I-messages. Tell him how much you miss him and how, more than anything else, you want to feel close to him. Talk about the ways in which his separateness from you hurts your feelings about yourself as a woman. Don't criticize him or talk about his inadequacies. Just talk about you. Make sure he really gets how bad you feel about your sexual relationship. If you tiptoe around the subject, he might not understand the seriousness of the situation. Here's a letter from a guy who missed the point and now suffers because his wife has chosen to have an affair:

Please do something to tell your husband how serious this is before you complicate matters with an affair. Do everything in your power to explain to him where you are headed if something does not change. I know you feel like you have already, but you have to get his attention. Having been there, I don't think you have his attention yet.

He needs to know how important sex is to you and that your marriage is in serious jeopardy. Give it to him straight.... "You are considering finding someone else who will give you the love you deserve" if the two of you cannot get it together. Please, for your sake as well as his, give him every opportunity to change. If he can't or is unwilling to change and you will know in your heart that you tried everything you could to make the marriage work, then separate.

I'd give anything to be able to spend the rest of my life explaining the depth of my feelings to my wife. It would take me that long to beg her forgiveness and to apologize for the idiot that I was. She tried, but I did not understand. I do now! Ironically, just before we split up, we found our sex life. With better understanding on both sides, we were compatible, and it was great! It appears, however, that it was too late.

After you're done expressing your feelings, ask for what you want; don't complain. Review the goals you set in Chapter 6, and tell him specifically what he could do to help you feel better about your sex life. Talk in action-oriented terms. For instance, tell him, "I know you haven't been up for having sex recently, but I would really love it if you just hold me and kiss me a couple times a week when we're in bed. I would also be thrilled if you would help me have an orgasm once in a while, even if you don't want one yourself." That's specific. Tell him that he doesn't need to respond to you immediately; you just want to make certain that he knows how you feel. Then stop talking. Even if your husband doesn't respond or responds negatively, it doesn't mean that he won't take your feelings to heart. Just quietly observe what happens in the next few days and weeks and see if you've prompted a change.

Ask About Your Husband's Turn-Ons, and Then Turn It On!

You need to ask your husband what *specifically* turns him on. Even if he doesn't want sex as often as you, there must be things he likes about sex. Create a comfortable enough atmosphere to encourage him to fill you in about what excites him.

Once he tells you what turns him on, make mental notes. Don't judge, critique, or second-guess his responses. Take them at face value. Just remember that feelings aren't right or wrong; they just are. Some people really enjoy watching X-rated videos, while others find the thought upsetting. Some people like to play out kinky fantasies, while other, more inhibited people would find these sexual role plays distasteful. There are few universal rules about satisfying sex.

If he's been brave or invested enough to tell you what he likes, short of doing something illegal or illicit, see if you can do what he asks. If your husband tells you things he would like to do that don't really appeal to you, you need to find ways to compromise. Some solutions or compromises require more creativity than others, but with a little determination, you can create a win-win resolution. The important thing here is that your husband feels heard. If a man doesn't feel heard, he will shut down. Too often when men tell their wives about their turn-ons, women ignore or downplay the importance of what they're requesting.

For instance, I worked with men who have told their wives that they want them to wear thongs, shave their pubic hair, dress more seductively when they go out together, wear more (or less) eye makeup, get a new hair style, and so on, and women underestimate the importance of these requests. Some women have told me that they think their husbands are being controlling, that they should be able to be or dress any way they want. Is that right? Well, certainly, that's right. But if your man is sharing information about what gets his juices flowing, if you completely disregard his wishes, he'll stop talking. He'll figure, "What's the point?" Let him know that his feelings matter.

> Desire (for me) is only minimally based on body shape. I have taken great care to convince my wife that a smile works a lot better than makeup/perfume/clothes/etc. Now, my wife rarely wears makeup, almost exclusively to the more formal events. This is great for me. Makeup tends to rub off on me, and I find it irritating. Perfume is exciting for about five minutes, then starts to drive me away in an effort to get some air I can breathe. I enjoy her own scent more than any perfume. She doesn't use perfume anymore, and I like that a lot.

Of course, if your husband is requesting something that violates your personal moral code, that's a different story. I worked with a couple in a long-term marriage where the man said that the only way he could feel really turned on was if she agreed to having a threesome with another woman. She desperately wanted to please her husband, but the thought of having three-way sex positively violated everything in which she believed. She refused. Her marriage suffered. However, this is an extreme case. What your husband needs or wants to boost his desire may fit well within your values. And if it's a stretch, try to find a way to compromise.

Ask About Potential Turnoffs

In addition to asking your husband what turns him on, you should also inquire as to what turns him off; it's important to know what you need to do more of *and* what you need to do less of. I know it's hard to ask, "Is there anything you'd prefer I stop doing or that I do differently?" but it's essential that you do.

Dale rarely had sex with his wife, Cora, because he felt so turned off by the words she used to initiate sex: "Do you want to do me?" Dale felt she sounded very self-centered and cold. He said he felt a sinking feeling in his stomach every time she asked him The Question.

When Dale shared what he was really feeling about Cora's words, she was shocked. She had no idea that he had such a negative response to her invitation for sex. She thought it sounded "flirty," but not to Dale. So I had Dale share with Cora what he would like her to say instead. He said, "I'd like it if she asked, 'Do you want to fool around?' or 'Do you want to make love?' I would be okay with her not saying anything and just start rubbing my thighs or kissing my neck. I would definitely feel more excited."

Dale's comments caught Cora by surprise; she found it hard to believe that a few simple words would have so much power, but she was more than willing to try a new approach.

At first when Cora varied her approach to Dale, it was a little awkward because it was something they both consciously decided to do after talking to me. It didn't just happen naturally. However, they started making light of it and ended up laughing as a result. Humor became their aphrodisiac.

Another man told me,

My wife has a higher sex drive. However it is at inappropriate times—right when I walk in the door after a hard day of work. She has three teenage kids from a previous marriage, and I'm uncomfortable with the way she is when I get home. Then when the kids go to their father's house (every two weeks for two weeks), she has no sex drive. She spends her time playing video games, smoking, and drinking beer. So, yes, my sex drive has become lower. I have actually told her about my feelings, but she just dismisses them as nonsense, and that makes me feel unheard. This is a vicious cycle.

I would tell this woman to be more discreet as to when she "attacks" her husband. She should wait until they are alone. Plus, I would suggest that she cut back on her beer, cigarettes, and video games when she has her husband all to herself. I suspect he would be very receptive if she followed his advice.

Dr. Pat Love, author of *Hot Monogamy*, also suggests that you should respect your husband's sexual preferences. If a husband tells his wife that he feels more turned on after they take a shower or when the kids are asleep, she may think he is just putting things off so that sex never happens. But these may not just be excuses. Although you may have a hard time believing or understanding this because you are ready to go at the drop of a hat, your spouse may really need things to be a certain way in order to feel relaxed, comfortable, and turned on. As much as possible, you should try to honor these requests and not discredit your spouse when he is confiding in you about these preconditions.

One last thing: keep in mind that getting to know you and your spouse's sexual preferences is a lifelong endeavor. What works in your twenties probably won't work in your fifties. What works one week might not be as interesting the next. Life is about change. Always keep the lines of communication open. Don't assume you know anything about your husband's sexual interests just because he told you about them early in your marriage. Just keep talking.

The Nike Solution—"Just Do It"

I wish I had a dollar for each time a person in my practice said, "You know, I really wasn't in the mood for sex when we started out, but once I got into it, it really felt great. I had a great orgasm." I'd be independently wealthy by now. That's because this is an incredibly common situation. Lots of people with low sexual desire actually enjoy sex once they get started. They may have to clear out the mental clutter and slowly relax, but when they do, they tell me that sex is enjoyable. People can definitely jump-start their desire by getting their feet moving.

Tell your husband that you don't want to have intercourse, you just want to fool around—no pressure, no performance. Make sure you go slowly, giving him a chance to unwind, relax, and get lost in your touches. Stay away from his genitals until he gives you some indication that he's starting to get turned on. Let him pace you. If he seems excited, test the waters, and see if touching his penis feels good to him. If so, keep going. If not, hold back. Keep it to a pleasant, sensual touching session. In my experience, men are often surprised by how often their bodies respond even if their minds lag behind. It may surprise your husband to learn that for him, desire follows arousal rather than the other way around. It's certainly worth a try. Just do it.

Act As If

When we approach our spouse with an idea or a plan or behave in a certain way, we tend to envision what the reaction might be. We'll tell ourselves, "I feel certain he's going to go along with this," or "I just know that he's going to give me a hard time," or "I can predict that he's going to be nasty when I tell him _____" (fill in the blank). And you know what? Our expectations can have a tremendous impact on the results and responses we get. That's because we tend to behave in ways that broadcast our expectations in subtle yet definite ways. If we expect our spouse's criticism, we go into the situation with our dukes up, looking for signs that our husband is going to come down on us. Any small sign that he is less than welcoming becomes the center of our attention. Plus, our spouse is a thinking, feeling, sensing being. (Even if you aren't convinced of this, it's true.) He can pick up our concerns in our behavior. And then when he responds critically or defensively, we tell ourselves, "See, I knew I was right." You may be right, or it may be the self-fulfilling prophecy at work. I believe the latter.

And if my theory is right—"we think, therefore they are"—you can do a great deal to effect positive outcomes in your life. Ask yourself, "If I expect my husband to be kind, loving, positive_____, (again, fill in the blank), how would I act right now?" Act as if you believe in your heart of hearts that you're going to get the outcome you want, and behave toward your husband the way you would with this positive expectation in mind.

I was working with a woman, Betty, who complained that she and her husband, Ted, fought every night. Ted had become highly critical of her, and they hadn't made love in two months. Even prior to that, their lovemaking had been infrequent. Ted had stopped saying, "I love you," to Betty or showing any other signs of affection. According to her, Ted went to work, came home, ate dinner, and spent his night watching television.

Betty was very unhappy in the marriage and went to see a divorce attorney. However, prior to filing for divorce, she decided to seek help, and our work together began.

After a few sessions, a few things became clear. Betty expected every evening to be just like the last—conflict laden, unpleasant, and without affection. She barely said hello to Ted when he walked through the door for fear that he would bite her head off.

But as we talked, I discovered Betty and Ted had shared many good times together earlier in their relationship. Before their son was born, they were more sexual, loving, and light-hearted. Although Betty used to get up early in the mornings to make and eat breakfast with Ted, she had taken to sleeping in until the baby woke up. She used to make fancy bag lunches for Ted, but that stopped too. She stopped calling Ted at work just to say hello. She also stopped cooking elaborate dinners for them. Betty still did Ted's laundry, but left it on his side of the bed for him to put away himself. She was hoping he would appreciate her more if he noticed all that she used to do for him.

I quickly surmised what was happening in their marriage and why their sex life had dwindled. For one thing, Betty had only recently recovered from fluctuating hormones brought on by childbirth. She had been sleep deprived and physically exhausted. Plus, her son became the new love in her life. All the sweet little things she used to do for Ted were now directed toward their baby. Although the changes in her life were completely understandable, Betty was inadvertently giving Ted the message that he was no longer important to her. I know that wasn't true, or she wouldn't have been sitting in my office. I had to urge Betty to make her husband a bigger priority. It is my very strong belief that the best thing you can do for your kids is to put your marriage first.

I told Betty to try an experiment: do the things she used to do when she and Ted were getting along well and feeling more amorous. She was to treat Ted more like she did in the past and watch what happened. Although it took a couple of weeks for Betty to get the full effect of her experiment, this is what she said:

> I decided that I wasn't going to fight with him. When he started
> picking a fight, I just refused to participate. After a few times, I was

able to completely stop our arguments. He caught on to what I was doing, and once when *I* picked a fight, he just refused to fight with me. It was really great. I couldn't believe that my new method for getting along better was contagious!

You said I should start acting as if it were the old days, and so I did. I started making his lunches again. One night I made ribs for dinner, and he woke me up in the middle of the night to say, "Honey, those ribs you made were incredible. Thank you." I've been trying to be happier and more attentive when he's home too. We've been spending more time together at night. I quit ragging on him.

But the best thing has happened: we've been making love twice each week. That's about where we were before our son was born. He even told me that he loves me, something he hasn't said in a really long time. I feel like we're really back on track. My sister even noticed a big difference in us. She said we seem so much happier and more affectionate. Now I know that I can affect what happens in our marriage and our sex life, and I feel much more confident that our changes are going to stick.

Want to follow in Betty's footsteps? The next time you find yourself thinking negatively about how a situation may turn out, ask yourself:

- How would I approach this situation given my pessimism?
- What would I say? What would I do?
- How do I want the situation to turn out instead?
- How would I handle this situation differently if I were expecting good things to happen?

Get a clear image of how you would look and sound different to him. Could it be your tone of voice, facial gesture, body language that would change? What exactly could he sense about you that would be unusual? Once you get a picture of that in your mind, make a commitment to "act as if." Do it even if you don't fully believe it. Watch what happens next. Tamara is a forty-two-year-old woman who has been married for seventeen years to her husband, Brett. They have three children. Like many other couples, she remembers sex being a lot better and more experimental in the early part of their marriage. Tamara said, "The problem is the way we have sex. I am always ready for it. I think it is a huge part of our relationship and that some effort should be put into making it as good as it can be. Brett sees it as something that needs to be done, like scratching an itch. When he feels horny, the sole aim is to ejaculate. For me, I want to have fun, occasionally spending a few hours just enjoying touching, pleasuring, and foreplay, I suppose."

Tamara went on to tell me that they usually have sex when Brett wanted it—on weekday mornings—and that it was hurried, often leaving her unsatisfied. She admitted that Brett might spend a bit longer on weekends, but she felt it was under duress. Although she understood that men's physiology is such that they often are more interested in the morning, she still felt shortchanged because of his lack of enthusiasm. Plus, she thought Brett was judging her for wanting sex to be more experimental. These differences in their sexual relationship angered her so much that she decided to separate.

Brett and Tamara lived apart for a year. During that year, they both decided that they wanted to reconcile and work on their marriage. I knew that if Tamara approached Brett with her preconceived notions about his lack of interest in leisurely or innovative sex he would become defensive and resistant and fulfill her expectations. I told her: You are on the precipice of a new marriage with Brett. You have divorced your old marriage, and you can have a completely fresh start. Envision Brett being the man you want him to be sexually. Assume that he wants a rich and exciting sex life with you too. If you really believed in your heart of hearts that he wants a good sex life too, how might you approach him as you begin living together again?"

Here's what Tamara replied:

If I were expecting a positive outcome, here's what I could do differently. When Brett approached me in the morning, even if that's not my favorite time to get it on, I would be up for it and assume that even though we might not have hours to play together, he will still care about my having an orgasm and take a little more time to do what turns me on. I guess I would act as if I were very excited about sex, even if I wished it were happening a little later and lasting a little longer.

Also, if I approached him later in the day or wanted to try something more experimental or kinky, if he hesitated at first, rather than get my feelings hurt and retreat thinking, "Same old, same old," I could tell myself that he just needs a little more coaxing, seducing, convincing, and that once he's doing it, he'll like it. In other words, if I expected good things to happen, I would just keep going.

When Tamara put her plan into action, she reported that things were going much better with her new and improved "act as if" attitude.

I want to give you one more piece of advice about this "act as if" method. In the *Redbook*-Davis survey (Chapter 1), I noticed something interesting in the data: wives with high desire approached their husbands significantly less often than men with high desire approached their wives. And it's not because women with high desire are satisfied with a lot less sex than their high-desire male counterparts. I think it's because they expect their husband to turn them down. So tell yourself, "This time he's going to be turned on. He is going to want to make love." Ask yourself how you would approach your husband differently if you truly felt he would be responsive. Then cast your doubts to the wind and "act as if."

The Attraction Factor

Meet Lynn and Seth, a couple whose sex life had become practically nonexistent. Lynn was terribly upset about it and had no clue as to why Seth had been so distant. Finally Seth told Lynn that he felt turned off by the fact that she had gained thirty pounds after the birth of their second child. Lynn was a short woman, and thirty pounds must have made a tremendous difference in her appearance. What happened next turned things from bad to worse.

Lynn became defensive about her weight. She explained all the reasons she gained weight, including feeling down in the dumps due to his lack of help around the house and with the kids, having no free time to herself, his insensitivity about many issues in their relationship, and on and on. Then she began to confront him about his superficiality; she was upset about his not loving her for who she was inside. She reprimanded him for looking at just her shape, and not her spirit or her heart.

Although Lynn's reaction was completely understandable and even valid, her defensiveness shut down all communication between her and her husband. She invalidated his feelings. He vowed to share no more. This led to further hurt and distance in their marriage.

I have worked with many couples where one spouse has lost interest in sex because he or she no longer feels attracted to his or her mate. It may be due to a weight gain, sloppy appearance, poor hygiene, unhealthy habits such as smoking or drinking, or an unwillingness to care for oneself physically. Frequently when the spouse who is no longer attracted finally gets up the nerve to talk about it, he or she is met with defensiveness and anger:

> I would like to address the epidemic of low sex drive in married men. In my case, it has to do with the fact that my wife now weighs 50 pounds more than she did when she married me. She'll do many things to rekindle, i.e., candlelit dinners, bath sessions, Victoria's Secret, books on love tricks, etc.—all that effort and money on something that doesn't matter. Then she can say, "I've tried everything. He's simply lost interest in me. Boo-hoo." Well, why not LOSE SOME WEIGHT?! Can you imagine the turn-off when someone fifty or more pounds overweight dons a teddy and/or thong? But I don't dare breathe a word of that or even imply by actions that she weighs one ounce more than she did when I married her. Even if she asks, "Do you think I'm fat?" I don't fall for an honest answer. I just swallow and say what she wants to hear—the only answer she will accept. So when the subject of "rekindle the romance" comes up, how about a little directness?

If your husband has told you that he's not attracted to you or that he's unhappy about the fact that you're unfit, out of shape, or uncaring about your appearance in any way, whether you think it's enlightened, fair, right, or not, it just is. As I said earlier in this book, physical attraction is a very important part of desire. If you think that your husband should love the person within, I agree, he should, but he's having sex with the outside person as well. I know it may sound harsh for me to tell you these things and I know it may not be politically correct, but I'm in the business of helping people feel more love and connection; I'm not running for office. I want you to really be honest with yourself about your looks and the energy you put into being physically healthy and fit. And if your husband's feelings reflect even a morsel of truth, I know you can't be too happy with yourself either. That's what I discovered when I continued working with Lynn.

Lynn admitted that Seth wasn't the only one who was unhappy about the changes in her body; so was she. Lynn also admitted that it was one thing for her to feel that way about herself but completely another that Seth felt that way about her. I helped her get over the hurt, and once she did, Lynn agreed that it was time for her to get serious about getting her body back into shape. She decided to join a health club and start taking aerobic classes three times a week. Seth agreed to help more with the kids so that she could have the time she needed to devote to herself. Additionally, Lynn started a new, more healthful eating plan.

Although Lynn didn't become trimmer instantly (no one does), she immediately started to feel better about herself, and her improved self-esteem had a positive impact on their marriage as well. Seth appreciated the fact that Lynn had gotten serious about her fitness. He felt that for the first time, Lynn really cared about his feelings, and this made him feel closer to her. Although he didn't jump into bed with her instantly, they were making love again three weeks later, after a long sexual drought. And things went uphill after that.

I know that losing weight, getting fit, or becoming more physically appealing isn't easy for everyone, especially if you have an underlying physical condition; however, it's important that you truly hear what your husband has to say about his feelings toward you. Although some people can be unrealistic about their expectations, don't immediately assume that your husband is shallow or superficial because he wants you to change something about your looks. The mere fact that you are willing to consider his feelings may, as in Lynn and Seth's marriage, go a long way to bringing back the passion in your relationship.

Be willing to have a frank discussion about what turns your husband off about you at the moment. Make sure you are clear about what he would like you to change. Tell him that you'd like his help in turning over a new leaf. If he is skeptical because you've promised this in the past and didn't do it, or you've had your ups and downs in terms of successes, tell him that you understand why he is skeptical, but you would like his encouragement now nonetheless. Ask him to pay attention to the new things you'll be doing in the next few weeks to get things on track. Then whether he encourages you or not, start your new health regime and stick with it. It will take planning, time, and determination, but you will feel better about yourself as well.

The "Lovers Can't Be Married" or "Not-So-Hot Mama" Syndrome

Another reason men fall out of lust is that their partners' roles change, and with those changes go erotic tension. No one talks about this aspect of married life better or more illuminatingly than Dr. Esther Perel, author of *Mating in Captivity*, a truly provocative book. Perel writes of a couple where the man could no longer see his wife as desirable once they had children. He tells Perel, "I always considered myself to be very competent sexually. We kid around that we broke furniture when we first started dating; there was a lot of passion. I never looked at the kids as a defining moment in my life sexually, but obviously something switched somewhere deep inside . . . The whole physical thing was a little weird. I watched her give birth, twice, and I gotta say it was not so great for our sex life. . . . I became different with her, more cautious, not as free. I guess it stopped me from being aggressive or passionate or desiring her in that way—really giving myself to her, or taking her, when normally that's how we were together. It was definitely a shift." Perel suggests that this couple do anything that might "distinguish [the wife] from The Mother."

The wife took action by doing something that completely turned things around. She started giving her husband "an involved, prolonged, great blow job, but then told her husband that he would have to pay her 'a hundred bucks' if he wanted her to continue. This fantasy game catapulted her out of the Mother role and back into the femme fatale her husband knew her to be."

If your husband has had difficulty seeing you as erotic after you tied the knot or had children, rather than try to talk it out, try dreaming up some creative fantasy that casts you in a different and more daring or erotic light. You need to become the seductress again; your imagination can take you there.

I worked with a couple who had been married for three years. They both realized that the husband had been having a difficult time eroticizing his wife since the wedding, but more so in the past year. She was hot for sex, but he felt a bit turned off. I suggested that she get dressed up very seductively, go to a bar in their small town, and wait for her husband to find her there. He too was supposed to get spruced up and find the right bar by trial and error. Once there, he was to pretend to pick up this hot woman aka his wife. They loved this adventure and almost got kicked out of the bar for being "inappropriate." How very appropriate!

Spice Things Up

Okay, I'm going to level with you. Many men in my practice have confided in me that one of the main reasons they're not into sex is that they're bored. They don't tell their wives they're bored because they don't want to hurt their wives' feelings. Ask your husband if sex has became routine, and if so, what he would like to do for more excitement. I know that's a hard question to ask, and it might be unnerving to hear his answer, but until he gets it out in the open, nothing will change. Boredom is something that can be fixed.

> I've noticed I don't feel so sexed up anymore. Things between my wife and me have gotten ho-hum. I have no objections to her pleasing herself. She has hinted a few times, and my response has always been, "Can I watch?" but it almost never happens. I think it would make an interesting variant to add a little spice to the normal routine. I just don't feel like doing it the same old way anymore.

In addition to asking your husband what he'd like to do differently, you can take the initiative of trying new things yourself. Some women are shy about introducing new sexual activities into their lovemaking. If you have been one of those women, I suggest you push yourself. If your husband is bored, it will boost his desire, and you might just love it too.

Don't allow self-consciousness about your body to slow you down. You're not perfect, but no one else is either. If your husband has been wanting some novelty, he'll be excited with your creativity. If you're short of ideas, check out the resources in Chapter 13. There's no end to the new things you can try!

Keep in mind that it's not just the sex act itself that warrants some innovative moves; the seduction process sets the tone:

- Tell him you are not wearing panties. Whispering this to him in public is especially good.
- Wear a blouse or shirt that hangs open when you bend over, and flash him.

When you are at home you can be even more direct, especially if you have no kids around. Even if you have kids, you can find a moment here or there.

- Walk into the room naked from the waist up or the waist down.
- Without warning, while he is watching, lift your shirt, massage your breasts (getting your nipples erect is especially good), then lower your shirt, and go on as if nothing happened.

What you say can also affect him. No doubt these sound corny to you, but try some and see what happens. By the way, most men are grabbed by "slang" terms, so if you don't have a problem using them in their sexual way, try it.

- "I've been thinking about your penis all day."
- "I was thinking about having sex with you, and now I'm all wet."

You can also arouse him by touching him. His penis is the center of his sexuality, so go there if you can.

- Feel him up at a stop light.
- Sit across from him at dinner, slip off your shoe, and massage his crotch with your foot.

Paul and Lori Byerly, founders of the Web site www.themarriagebed .com, have some fun ideas about boosting your husband's desire. Visit their . Web site for a racy list of suggestions!

Boost Your Sexual IQ

Many sexual problems are caused by a low sexual IQ. If one of the reasons you're slow to experiment sexually or you're missing the mark with your husband is that you're not confident about your knowledge about sex, you're not alone. Remember, we're not born knowing how to please our partners or to have great sexual experiences. In addition to asking your husband about his particular pleasures, there are many excellent resources available to help you learn more about having great sex. Your husband knows what he likes, but he might not be aware of new and exciting possibilities he's never tried before. You can lead the way. Check out the Resources in Chapter 13 for books, tapes, and seminars that might enlighten both of you. You can learn about sex in the privacy of your own home with many of these products.

I can't say enough about the importance of seeking help from a certified sex therapist if you need it. Since good sex therapists are also sex educators, sex therapy can be one of the most enlightening experiences you will ever have.

After experimenting with the sexy solutions in this chapter, I trust you've found some helpful advice and that things are looking up. Now here's your challenge—keep it up! That's what the next chapter is all about.

CHAPTER TEN

Keeping It Up

It's great that you have gotten this far, and I hope you and your husband have seen improvements in your sexual relationship. Besides having more frequent intercourse, I hope you are touching nonsexually, flirting, being more playful, and feeling like intimate partners again. I think it's great that you have been willing to work so hard to feel more connection and intimacy in your marriage. You should definitely take some time out to congratulate yourself in your stick-to-itiveness and your search for solutions. I'm so glad you didn't just throw in the towel. The changes in your marriage have taken time, energy, patience, and great sensitivity, but I assume you'll agree that it's certainly been worth the effort.

But don't get too comfy soaking up the good feelings between you. I've seen too many couples assume that once things are better, they are going to stay better. Yes, you should enjoy your luscious moments together, but you really must have a plan in place to keep the changes going.

It took work for the two of you to recharge your sex life, and you will have to continue to do what has been working if you want to continue to have good results. The first part of your maintenance program is to identify specifically what you both have been doing that has been working.

Next you will need to recognize the signs when you and your husband might be moving in the *wrong* direction. You might be thinking, "Of course, I'll know when things are deteriorating: sex will start being a problem again." As you should know by now, "sex will start being a problem again" is not a clear enough signpost. You will need to be able to identify *specifically* what will be going on in your marriage that will make you think, "Time to do something about this." I'm going to help you decipher what constitutes a backslide in your marriage so that when it happens, there will be no question that it's time for action. And you and your husband should also have a specific plan for what to do when you start to notice that things are slipping.

As you can probably tell, I think it's absolutely essential that you not take your positive changes or each other for granted. The more you know about preventing relapse and maintaining change, the more you'll stay on the passion track.

WHAT'S BEEN WORKING?

Throughout this book, I've been preaching, "If it works, don't fix it; do more of it." And that's what I want you to do right now. Get a pen and paper and write down your responses to the following questions:

- Think back to a time when your sex life wasn't very satisfying to you. Briefly describe what was happening then. Write down what you and your husband were doing (or not doing) and the feelings you had at the time.

- Think about what's been better in the past days, weeks, or months. Describe the improvements in action-oriented terms. What are you both doing now that you didn't do so much before? Also include how your feelings have changed for the better.

- How do you think your husband would respond to the previous two questions? You don't need to ask him to do this with you, but you can if you'd like. The point is for you to become clear about what's different in your marriage now that things are better.

- How do you approach your husband differently to bring about these positive changes? What have you been doing or saying to create more responsiveness in him? What has been working?

- What would your husband say you've been doing differently that he appreciates?

- How has your husband been treating you differently that has motivated you to stick to the positive ways of interacting?

ARE WE SLIPPING?

Your sex life is going along swimmingly. You're touching and kissing more, there is a more relaxed feeling between you, and you're even having more frequent and enjoyable intercourse. You assume it will be easy to tell when things are going downhill. Will it be the time you make love and nothing seems to go right? What if he loses his erection, or you don't have an orgasm? Will it be when you hit a two-week sexless period when, until then, you've been making love once or twice a week? Will you be concerned when, after months of his agreeing to be more adventurous, your husband wants to have sex only in the missionary position again? Or if he tells you three times in a row that he's not interested in having sex?

Although what constitutes backsliding for one couple is entirely different than it is for another, I want to caution you about a few things. Life isn't perfect. Sex isn't perfect. Marriage isn't perfect. (Am I telling you anything you didn't already know?) But when I work with couples, something interesting happens. After they've endured painful times, and life begins to be happier and more fulfilling, they assume or hope that's how things will always be. But everything in life is subject to ebb and flow, including your sex life. The worst mistake you and your husband can make is to have unrealistic expectations about your sexual relationship.

Even people who are really happy with their love lives admit that sex isn't always great. Orgasms don't necessarily happen every time. You won't always feel close and connected when you make love. His penis might go limp from time to time. He will be preoccupied and totally disinterested in physical contact occasionally. That exciting position you tried last week produced a ho-hum effect today. In short, despite what you see in the movies or read about in romance novels, sex isn't hot all the time, no matter how much you love your spouse, how much you've changed, how attractive you think you are or he is, or even how much you want it to be. Sometimes sex is just okay, unsatisfying, or even nonexistent.

You've got to learn to not overreact and start thinking that your marriage and sex life is crumbling if you have a few bad sexual episodes or feel disconnected for a while. You need to tell yourself, "Michele warned me that this is going to happen, that all couples have ups and downs and that I shouldn't panic." That should be your mantra. Don't make a big issue out of a passing condition. It will only make matters worse.

However, it's important for you to identify what *will* signify a significant step backward so that you and your husband can recognize it and nip it in the bud. Here are some questions to ask yourself:

- Given how much better our lives have been going recently, what would have to happen that would make me think, "Oh-oh! We're going downhill"? What would my husband and I be doing differently that would be a cause for concern? What would be different about our sexual relationship or marriage that would really worry me?
- How could I tell the difference between things that are off once in a while versus things that are happening that should raise a red flag? What specifically will be different about those times when we need to do something to fix it?
- What would your husband say would be a sign that things are slipping?
- Between the two of you, who do you think would be the first to notice that things are going backward?

I worked with Faith and Zach for several months. Faith's complaint was that Zach frequently turned down her requests for sex but she would often "catch" him masturbating instead. This hurt and infuriated her. She couldn't understand why Zach would prefer his hand over her, and she felt both exasperated and dejected. When she confronted him with her feelings, he said very little and promised he would try harder to please her. Yet the pattern continued.

In our work together, I learned that Zach rarely talked to Faith about his feelings about sex. He loved oral sex and felt that Faith wasn't interested in pleasing him that way. He also wanted her to be more creative and willing to dress up and role-play. He often fantasized about her dressing up like a hooker and seducing him. But he never told her that. In fact he failed to mention that he was dissatisfied at all. He just avoided sex because, in his mind, it had become routine. He found more excitement in masturbating to girlie magazines.

When Zach was more open with Faith about his desires in our sessions, he was surprised to find out that Faith was completely willing to be more playful and adventurous. In the rare times when Zach had not rejected Faith, she felt too insecure to try anything new. She was just glad that Zach had agreed to have sex. Now that she knew more about what he really wanted, she was eager to please him in new, and even "kinky," ways.

It wasn't long before they returned and reported that things were going much better for them sexually. Because Faith was "doing all the right things," Zach was not only more responsive when she approached him, he was approaching her. Faith said that it felt "just like the old days, before they had kids." For weeks, they kept up their newfound enthusiasm for experimentation, and it was mutually satisfying.

Several weeks later, Faith came to see me alone. She wanted to check something out with me. Although sex was still good between them, Faith was concerned because Zach would masturbate from time to time. She worried that he would return to using masturbation as a replacement for lovemaking.

I asked Faith how often he masturbated and she said, "Once or maybe twice a week . . . that I know about." And then I asked, "How often did he masturbate in the past when you were hardly making love at all?" She replied, "I think he was masturbating every day." Ultimately I wanted to know whether despite Zach's occasional masturbation she believed that their sex life was still on track. And without hesitation, she said yes.

We talked a while about how some people really enjoy masturbation even when they have healthy and loving sexual relationships with their spouses; one activity does not necessarily preclude the other. I wondered if she had thought about incorporating masturbation into their lovemaking, and she hadn't—but she was certainly willing to give it a try.

I also said, "I can see why you might have been concerned. Some of what was happening in the past when things weren't going well appeared to be happening again. But when we take a closer look at your situation, despite his enjoying masturbating once in a while, you are still having a good time with each other sexually. It's great that you checked it out with me, but from where I stand, it's not a problem."

I asked what would have to happen for her to be convinced that things are truly sliding, and she said, "Since we've worked with you, Zach has realized the importance of discussing his honest feelings about sex with me, and he's continued doing that. As long as I know what he's thinking so I can try to please him, we'll be okay. If he clams up and pulls away and we start having sex only twice a month, that will be a sign I need to do something . . . pronto."

What separates the winners from the losers when it comes to making positive changes in life isn't how often you take a step backward, it's how quickly you get yourself back on track. If things are offtrack, don't waste time berating yourself or your husband or analyzing things to death. Don't feel sorry for yourself. Just pick yourself up, dust yourself off, and do what you must to get things back on track.

A CALL TO ACTION

Once you've decided that things truly have taken a turn for the worse, you need to take swift action. Review the techniques and solutions you discovered along the way; chances are, you just stopped doing them. Reinstitute those solutions. Don't spend too much time talking about it; just do your part. If that doesn't work, talk to your husband about your perception. See if he too has noticed things sliding. If he agrees, discuss what each of you needs to do to get out of the doldrums.

Dr. Barry McCarthy, sex therapist and author, offers couples many great ideas for preventing relapse. According to McCarthy, the more ways to maintain an intimate sexual connection, the easier to avoid relapse. Here are a few of his suggestions:

1. Every six months have a formal follow-up meeting by yourselves or with a therapist, to ensure that you remain aware and do not slip back into unhealthy sexual attitudes, behaviors, or feelings. Set a new couples goal for the next six months.

2. Every four to eight weeks, plan a sensual pleasuring session or a playful erotic session with a prohibition on intercourse.

3. The importance of setting aside quality time, especially intimacy dates and a weekend away without children, cannot be emphasized enough.

4. There is not one "right way" to be sexual. Each couple develops their unique style of initiation, pleasuring, erotic scenarios and techniques, intercourse, and after-play. Rather than treating your couple sexual style with benign neglect, be open to modifying or adding something new or special each year.

5. Develop a range of intimate, pleasurable, and erotic ways to connect, reconnect, and maintain connection, such as:

> Affectionate touch
> Nongenital sensual touch
> Playful touch
> Erotic, nonintercourse touch
> Intercourse

If, after talking to your husband about your perception, he disagrees, you can sit back for a while and think about whether you're overreacting. Even if he didn't acknowledge or agree with what you said, it doesn't mean he won't think about it. He will. Then watch his behavior over the next few days. You might notice his coming toward you.

But, if your husband doesn't acknowledge a problem, you may be reverting to your old patterns. Ask him to get some help with you. Tell him that you've been feeling so great about your sex life, and you don't want to lose it. Ask if he would consider seeing a therapist as "love insurance." If he agrees, schedule an appointment, or consider calling a Sex-Starved Marriage coach from my office (page 210) or 800-664-2435 or 303-444-7004. But beyond that, if he's still stubbornly resisting your efforts to get things back on track, it's time for you to read the next chapter: "When He Resists."

CHAPTER ELEVEN

When He Resists: Sex 911

I am at my wit's end. I have been married for five years. We got married after about three months of knowing each other and having a whirlwind romance. I was the happiest I had ever been in my life. Two years into our marriage, my husband just stopped wanting sex. We went from having really great sex two or three times a week to about once every six weeks. And when we have sex, it's like he's somewhere else. Something is wrong. I'm lonely, angry, hurt. I have tried everything I can think of to reach him. I have tried again and again to get him to tell me what's wrong, but he just won't talk. I ask him to get help and he won't. He won't do one thing differently to change his behavior. I'm still young, and we don't have kids. I don't know how much longer I can take this. I love my husband, I want my marriage, but I won't go on like this forever. I'm seriously thinking of leaving. I just don't know what else to do.

It's my sincere hope that "When He Resists" will be the world's least-read chapter. However, realist that I am, I know that not all women will be successful in improving their sex lives. Some women will be on cloud nine, others will notice minor improvements, and still others will feel as stuck as they were when they began reading the book. I hope that's not you, but if it is, I want to help you sort out what to do next.

In the same way that a car mechanic goes through a series of tests to eliminate potential causes of the problem one at a time, we'll go through a troubleshooting checklist one step at a time. By the time we're done, I hope you'll have a better understanding of what you need to do next.

Before you read on, I want to remind you of my bias. I'm a diehard marriage saver. I really believe in my heart of hearts that most marriages can, and *should*, be saved. I feel certain, without even knowing you, that most of the problems you're having are fixable with the right help. It's always my preference to help people rediscover the passion in their marriage so they don't have to divorce and dissolve their families. So this chapter is geared to helping you make sure you leave no stone unturned before deciding that your marriage is dead. I have to believe that you agree with me about this, or you wouldn't be fighting so hard to make your marriage sexier and more loving. I think we're on the same team. So here goes.

HAVE YOU GIVEN A PARTICULAR APPROACH ENOUGH TIME?

Once you had chosen an approach and tried it out, how long did you wait before you determined that it wasn't working well? How long did you wait before you thought to yourself, "This is baloney; he's not going to change"? Many times I work with people who are so eager to make things better that they become impatient when trying a new approach. They wait several days, and if nothing changes, they assume the approach isn't working, become frustrated, and fall back into old patterns.

When this happens, I encourage people to slow down. I ask that they wait at least a few weeks to see if their new strategy is making a difference. In fact, sometimes it takes longer than that. The key is to wait several weeks—without hinting that you're waiting for something or hovering over him too conspicuously—and just quietly observe. Don't comment, and don't get angry; just watch. If, after two or three weeks, nothing changes at all, it's time to try a different approach.

HAVE YOU BEEN FLEXIBLE AND TRIED SEVERAL DIFFERENT APPROACHES?

Throughout this book I have told you that if what you're doing isn't work-ing, do something different. There are so many ideas in these chapters that it's impossible to try them all, but before vetoing any particular technique because you assume it won't work, try being a little more open-minded and experiment; go a little outside your comfort zone. It might not work, but you've got nothing to lose, and you want to be able to say to yourself that you've been flexible and open-minded. Go back and review my sug-gestions, and see if you glossed over any of them too quickly.

HAVE YOU TRIED A MARRIAGE EDUCATION CLASS?

If you haven't been able to resolve your issues, I'd be willing to bet that it's because you and your husband are either lacking communication skills, or you might have a low sexual IQ. It's nothing to be ashamed about; many couples don't have the sexual skills necessary to get their sexual relation-ship back on track.

A good, solid, marriage education class can really help. And if you and your husband are a bit on the squeamish side when it comes to doing "group stuff," don't worry. Marriage education classes aren't like group therapy. In fact, in most of those seminars, you and your husband will not have to publicly disclose any personal information. You will be "students," learning skills and practicing them—just the two of you. In the resource chapter of the book, I give information about some excellent skill-building seminars (page 216).

HAVE YOU ASKED YOUR SPOUSE
TO GO FOR THERAPY?

I know this is a touchy subject. In our *Redbook*-Davis poll, it was clear that low-desire men aren't crazy about seeking help, but if you haven't already, it's time to insist that he go with you. Suggest that you will either allow him to choose the therapist or you will. You really need him to go for at least a few sessions to see if he can get something out of it. If he hates it, tell him you would be willing to try a different therapist, but you are certain that you both need help. Tell him that it's not about fixing him; you have a problem too, and you want to work together on this issue. If he agrees even halfheartedly, schedule an appointment.

Make sure your therapist is experienced in marital or sex therapy. Too often therapists say they do marriage therapy just because they have a couple sitting in the office. This is rubbish. Marital therapy requires very different skills from doing individual therapy. Individual therapists usually help people identify and process feelings. They assist them in achieving personal goals.

Couples therapists need to be skilled at helping people overcome the differences that naturally occur when two people live under the same roof. They need to know what makes a marriage tick. They help people learn how to communicate and negotiate better. It's about relationship improvement rather than personal growth. A therapist can be very skilled as an individual therapist and be clueless about helping couples change. For this reason, ask your therapist about his or her training and experience in both marital and sex therapy.

Sex therapy is a particular specialty, and a licensed sex therapist must have taken certain courses. It's a good idea to speak to someone who is skilled in sex therapy. Chapter 13 provides information on finding the right therapist.

In choosing a therapist, here are some things to keep in mind:

- ***Choose a therapist who is goal oriented.*** Make sure your therapist asks you about your goals in the first session. Make certain you, your husband, and the therapist know what you want to accomplish.

Don't make sessions a rehashing of how your week went. It might be fun to have an outlet for complaining but it won't be productive. Know what you want to improve, and make sure you're working with someone who keeps you on track with those goals.

- *Therapy is meant to be a collaborative process.* Although the therapist has expertise, you and your husband are the experts in your own lives. You both should feel respected, heard, and appreciated. The therapist should not take sides or lean too hard on either one of you. You both need to feel comfortable with this person and need to believe that he or she is truly an ally for your marriage.

- *Your therapist should instill hope.* People generally don't seek therapy until they are so down in the dumps that hope dangles by a thread. Hopelessness is the real cancer in marriage. A good therapist is a hope monger. If your therapist is very skilled, no matter how long you've been experiencing your sexual problems, she or he will not be discouraged. In fact, your therapist should have skills to help you relate in new ways and feel more optimistic about the possibilities of change pretty rapidly.

- *The therapist should focus on your strengths and resources rather than spend long periods of time dissecting your deficits or what isn't working.* The most efficient way to rebuild a marriage is to focus on couples' strengths and resources and help them expand their assets. No matter how long you've been at odds, I want to remind you that you both have untapped skills. Your therapist should help you identify these hidden strengths and offer creative advice about how to put these strengths to use.

WHAT IF HE WON'T GO TO THERAPY?

It's entirely possible that no matter what you've tried or how clear you've been about the importance of seeking help, your husband won't budge. Then what do you do? Here are some last-resort suggestions.

Give an Ultimatum

Personally, I'm not big on ultimatums. Nobody likes being forced to do something. But there are people who won't change until they really feel that the demands are serious. Change forces people to move outside their comfort zones, and lots of people won't do that until they have something to lose. In other words, the anticipated discomfort of changing pales in comparison to the anticipated discomfort of losing something.

If you are at the point that you're ready to leave your marriage if your husband doesn't change, you might consider an ultimatum. However, I highly recommend that you not use it as a threat that you're not willing to follow through on. He might call your bluff, and then what are you going to do? Don't rely on being able to "take it back." Once you draw a line in the sand, mean it. You should intend to follow through with your consequences if your husband doesn't comply.

If you are truly at the end of your rope and seriously considering leaving your marriage if things don't improve, it may be time to get really tough. You can tell him face-to-face or write him a letter. Let him know that you love him and you want your marriage to work, but that you are desperately unhappy with the way things are going. You feel as if every day out of your life when you're not close and connected is another day lost. Tell him that you don't want to live like this any longer and that you want to get help for your marriage. Insist that he join you. You know that he probably won't like the idea, but tell him that he needs to do it for you, your marriage, and your children if you have them. Tell him that you are giving him a few days to think over his response very carefully. But in all fairness, you want him to know that if he chooses not to work on your marriage or provide any solutions to the ongoing stalemate, you will have to leave the marriage.

Of course, you don't have to use my words, but you should include the ideas I've suggested. Then wait a few days and see what happens. If he doesn't say anything, ask. If he says he'll go with you, get an appointment promptly. If he says, "Forget it," thank him for his response, and tell him you will begin to make your own plans. If he asks what you mean, tell him that you're not exactly sure yet. End the conversation.

Go to Therapy Alone

I am a strong believer that you should seek therapy by yourself even if your husband won't go. You can learn a lot about yourself and may even get additional ideas about how to lure your husband to therapy down the road. Just go; it will be good for you. Find a therapist who believes in marriage; the last thing you want from a therapist is someone who, after hearing about your situation, says, "Why would you want to put up with that?" You don't need to pay a professional for that sort of advice; your friends and family will be happy to offer it to you for free.

Leave

Since you are the expert on you, if you believe that you have nothing left to give your marriage, you can always leave. You know this is not my general recommendation, particularly when there are children involved, but it certainly is an option. Just make sure you've carefully considered all aspects of your future life, the kids, financial matters, coparenting, custody and visitation schedules, being single again, and so on. Really think things through. Divorce is (usually) forever. And then of course, read my book *The Divorce Remedy*. Don't leave home without it.

Stay and Be Miserable

Another option to consider is staying in your marriage and changing nothing. By changing nothing, you can ensure that you'll stay miserable. Although you will think that this choice sounds absurd and in fact doesn't even sound like a real choice, it is. Many women choose this option—they do it unwittingly, but they choose it nonetheless.

Stay and Focus on the Strengths in Your Marriage

Stay and develop a Zen-like detachment from the problem. You assume that your husband won't change, and instead of taking it personally and focusing your entire existence on the unhappiness you feel because your sexual relationship is less than it could or should be, you decide to accept and find peace with what is. You remind yourself that everyone is a package deal; there are things you love about that person and things you really can't stand about that person. You can trade your spouse for another one, and while you will undoubtedly resolve some problems, you will be faced with a whole new set of problems.

Patricia couldn't wait to divorce her low-drive husband because she had met the sexiest, most passionate, romantic man at work. This man made no bones about the fact that he was crazy about Patricia. He knew that she and her husband were unhappy and he wanted her to leave her husband so that they could be together. He wined and dined her. They flirted after hours. He kissed her passionately, which led to a sizzling hot affair. She knew she needed to get divorced. And she did.

Patricia and her coworker started dating seriously. It didn't take long before some of the heart-throbbing passion when they were together started to subside. In addition, after seven months into the relationship, Patricia learned that her new boyfriend had a few other women on the side. Apparently this guy's passion wasn't just for Patricia; his passion runneth over. Patricia was devastated by the news of his philandering and wondered why he wasn't as loyal and faithful as her ex-husband had been through all the years of their marriage. Granted, her ex wasn't the sexiest man in the world, but at least he was there for her. Patricia felt deeply saddened as she contemplated the choice she had made to end her marriage.

So what could Patricia have done differently? I will be the first to say that sex and physical closeness are a foundation of a loving, passionate marriage. That's why I wrote this book. But I want to tell you that sex isn't everything. It's important, but it's not everything.

If you love your spouse and want to stay married even if your sex life isn't great, you can consciously decide to focus on what's good about your marriage and for the most part let go of the rest. Here's an example of a woman who had been less than satisfied with her sexual relationship, but when she got an attitude change, her whole life lifted. And her marriage is sweeter than ever.

My husband, Cory, and I have been married for just over six years. Our sexual problems began almost immediately after the wedding, not because of lack of interest on either side but because I was taking a form of birth control that caused near-constant menstrual spotting. During what should have been our "honeymoon phase," my physical issue made sexual intimacy very difficult. I remember Cory being very patient, but I was extremely frustrated. Once I switched to a different birth control medication that regulated my periods, I was primed and ready to go, but it seemed like Cory had become accustomed to life with little or no sex (we had sex about once a month at this point). This confused me because before we got married, he couldn't wait to tear off my clothes.

We had a lot of tearful (on my part) discussions about how important I felt sex was to our relationship. I believed that if we missed the boat so early, we might never establish a strong sexual bond and could end up in a "roommate" marriage like my parents had. Even though all the other elements in our relationship were going well, I was extremely worried about this area of our life, and unfortunately, this concern overshadowed many of the positives.

Cory has a very responsible and high-paying position . . . and by his own admission, he often inadvertently allows his preoccupation with work and other outside concerns to spill over into our relationship. His ruminations would keep him from even thinking about sex with me, let alone acting on it. A lot more tearful discussions ensued, usually with me going to bed frustrated and unsatisfied and him promising to "keep working on it."

Although the frequency of our sexual encounters has not increased dramatically, the quality is, and always has been, excellent (the primary reason why I want more of it!). When my focus shifted away from quantity to quality, I believe our sex life improved considerably. I still do desire more sex than my husband does, but we've learned to communicate more openly and in a way that is less emotional so that sexuality is not a battleground anymore. I have become more comfortable with making sexual overtures (and not taking it so personally when he is tired, etc.), and this has taken some of the pressure off him being the sole initiator of sex. In the same way we had to negotiate the division of labor for household chores, we've had to navigate what sexuality would mean for us and to stop comparing ourselves to some illusionary ideal.

Within the past year, for example, I have begun seeing our customary hello and goodbye hugs and kisses as an integral part of our sexual relationship. I now see sexuality as a continuum instead of an end point, and as such, sex is much more than just intercourse. For his part, Cory has worked very hard on not allowing his outside worries to interfere with our intimacy, and I feel that he is much more attentive sexually as a result.

If I had any advice for other women dealing with similar issues, it would be to RELAX (which is easier said than done, I know). Focus on what's good about your relationship, even if those things are outside the bedroom. My husband and I have a wonderful relationship, and we enjoy a respectful and fun friendship that is the envy of many of our friends. We both believe we are "mates for life," and we have a strong sense of security in our marriage. As we have learned to shift our focus away from the things that were going wrong, it's been easier to relax into the relationship and to remember the unique, exciting aspects of each other that brought us together in the first place.

Don't you just love this woman? I do. If you want to stay in your less-than-perfect marriage (and whose isn't, by the way?), you can, and you can do it in style. But you have to change how you look at your husband, yourself, and your relationship. You really have to take an inventory of what you love about your husband and your marriage and see if you can focus on that and downplay the importance of having a robust sex life. I'm not saying you *should* do this; all I'm saying is that if you want to stay married, this is certainly a viable option. You always need to remember that no marriage is perfect. If your marriage is fairly sound except for your sex life, it may be too good to give up. If this seems like a decent option for you, ask yourself the following questions:

- What do I love about my husband?
- What strengths does he have as a person?
- Is he a good father?
- Are we good friends?
- Other than our fighting about sex, do we get along fairly well?
- What does he give me that I would miss if he weren't in my life?
- In what ways, other than physically, do I feel connected to him?

Besides focusing on the strengths in your marriage, if you choose to stay and make yourself happier, you will need to focus on *you*. You will need to build into your life lots of activities and people who will help enrich you. Meet and hang out with new friends. Cherish your relationships with them. Find new interests. Take a new class or change jobs. Take a trip with just you and the kids. Introduce novelty into your life. Break old habits and patterns. Stretch yourself outside your comfort zone. Volunteer some-where. Go to (or go back to) church or temple. Find ways to find peace within yourself.

And one more thing: stay sexy. Just because your husband is not oozing with sexuality doesn't mean that you're not a sexy woman. Continue to do the things you like to do to feel good about your sexual identity. Work out, dress up, and look hot. Flirt if you want, but I don't recommend infidelity. It's a short-term solution with long-term disastrous repercussions. But there's nothing wrong with fantasizing or satisfying yourself sexually and really allowing yourself to get into it. Just do it without anger or resent-ment. Do it for yourself. Feeling sexy is a do-it-yourself job anyway. Don't resign from the job simply because your husband is taking a sabbatical. He may not be interested, but that says nothing about you and your vibrancy as a woman. You're hot, or you wouldn't be reading this book.

But what should you do if, even after putting this chapter into action, your husband still is missing in action sexually? Read the next chapter. It will help you sort out whether some issues not yet addressed in this book may be lurking in your marriage.

CHAPTER TWELVE

When Low Desire
Isn't Really Low Desire

To a sex-starved wife, the only thing worse than a husband with little or no sexual desire is a husband who truly is interested in sex—but not with her. That's a double blow. Unfortunately, many husbands who reject their wives' sexual advances don't do so because of low sexual desire, but because they are finding other outlets for sexual satisfaction. What are they doing? They're engaging in self-sex—or masturbating. They're turning to the Internet. They're having emotional and sexual affairs. They're sexually addicted. And last, but certainly not least, there are men who are questioning their sexual identity. They're wondering whether they are in fact heterosexual. Let's take a closer look at each of these obstacles to a satisfying sexual relationship in marriage.

MASTURBATION

We have been married for ten years. For eight of those years, I have noticed his drive lessening. The thing that really upsets me is my husband masturbates more than we have sex. We average having sex maybe once every two weeks. I would be happy with twice a week. More would be nice, but I could be happy with twice. I could be lying next to him, and he has gotten up and masturbated. We have been home alone, and he has gotten up and masturbated. I drop the kids off at school and am home shortly to our house that we have all alone. And he has masturbated in that short time I was away. So I think, How can he prefer his male hand to the feeling of a woman?

Here are the facts: masturbation—touching your genitals for sexual arousal and/or achieving orgasm—is normal. Little children do it. Teens do it. Men do it. Women do it. Single people do it. Married people do it. In short, most people do it. It is said that 98 percent of people masturbate and the other 2 percent lie about it! Many young people's first sexual experience is through masturbation. Spouses often masturbate in each other's presence. All of this is normal and, for many people, very stimulating and satisfying. In fact, many experts agree that if people don't know how to achieve an orgasm through masturbation, they will not be able to coach their partners properly. So masturbation can be educational!

Masturbation becomes a significant problem if it detracts from sex with one's partner or if it's done compulsively and interferes with one's life. It is also problematic if it leads to a feeling of guilt or remorse. And of course, it goes without saying that masturbation is problematic, that is, criminal, when it's done in public.

My guess is that if you're reading this section about masturbation, you feel that your husband's interest in self-sex has dampened his desire for you. There are many reasons that a man would turn to masturbation as opposed to putting energy into having a healthy sex life with his wife. For starters most men learn about orgasms and sex through masturbation. They've had lots of practice. They know their bodies well and are often able to reach orgasm fairly easily. They don't need to know anything about pleasing a woman sexually, coordinating their pleasure with their partners, or how to deal with a moody woman who has just run short of estrogen.

Masturbation is a form of sexual expression that should not threaten or detract from marriage. However, if your husband is engaging in compulsive masturbation, it will leave him with little or no desire for you. But what's compulsive masturbation? Since there are no universal rules about a "normal" frequency for masturbation, it's somewhat difficult to define "compulsive" masturbation. In its extreme form, there are situations where some men masturbate hours and hours each week or to the point of self-injury. But things don't need to be that extreme for your marriage to be deeply affected by the behavior. Here's a definition I find helpful: if a behavior interferes with or becomes a replacement for one's personal, familial, or professional life, it's a problem. Additionally, when someone continually engages in sexual behavior despite negative consequences, such as compromised relationships, failed businesses, potential health risks, or a genuine desire to stop, it's also a problem. If this is happening in your marriage, you need to tackle this head-on.

Tell your husband about your concern. As always, discuss it in a loving way. Make sure he knows that you are not judging him for masturbating but that you're concerned that his focus on himself leaves him with little energy or motivation for sex with you. Ask him to tell you honestly whether there are things about your sexual relationship that he would like to be different. Tell him that you want to hear his thoughts and that you are willing to work on things with him. Reassure him that you are not expecting him to stop masturbating entirely; you just want to make sure that he has some reserves left over for you. He might be interested in incorporating masturbation into your lovemaking; let him know that that would be acceptable to you.

Also, many men masturbate when they feel insecure or uncertain about their ability to please their partner. They may experience erectile dysfunction or premature ejaculation. If this happens in your marriage, don't underestimate the impact of this problem on your husband's self-confidence. He may be masturbating rather than having sex with you because he fears failure. If you suspect that this might even be a possibility, talk about it openly. Let him know that you would love to be sexual without expectations of an orgasm. In other words, he doesn't have to perform. Review the information in Chapter 7 about overcoming sexual dysfunctions, and assure him that you are willing to work as a team to improve your sex life. The bottom line here is that you need to approach him in a nonjudgmental and supportive way. Remind him that professional help is available and highly effective.

EXCESSIVE INTERNET INVOLVEMENT

The Internet calls to mind how Charles Dickens began *A Tale of Two Cities*: "It was the best of times, it was the worst of times." Cyberspace has revolutionized our lives. Within seconds, we can have any kind of information we need or want at our fingertips. With the advent of the Internet, our world has shrunk; we can communicate with people across the globe as if they were living down the street. Anything we want to know, learn about, or investigate is there for the asking.

But there is a dark side to the Internet. Children are stalked by sexual predators; financial scams proliferate, victimizing unsuspecting and innocent people; and porn sites that can damage otherwise healthy marriages and families abound. The Internet offers easy, anonymous access for people seeking sexual pleasure, cyberaffairs, and illicit real-life relationships. Many people use the Internet as a substitute for real life, real relationship, and real sex.

My husband and I have been together close to 5 years now, married 3.5. He has NEVER exhibited a high sexual desire, which was foreign to me . . . I never had to ask for sex before, much less feel snubbed for it. On our first anniversary, I put my foot down and insisted on marriage counseling. We went, and wasted our time for well over a year . . . because my husband wasn't being honest with me or our counselor. He also continued to ignore sex and my requests for it. My instincts finally started screaming at me loud enough that I finally succumbed and installed a key logger on our home computer. I felt guilty and sneaky, but my instincts were telling me that things just weren't adding up. Less than ten hours after I installed the key logger, I had an answer. . . . He had a profile on Adult Friend Finders and had been communicating with women on it, viewing their photos/webcams and e-mail/chatting with them . . . all the while ignoring me and making me feel like I was pressuring him. The reality was . . . he was turning elsewhere.

A month ago, I found out the main reason I had been living as a sex-starved wife. My husband had actually been participating on adult Web sites where people go to hook up . . . or live out sexual fantasies. He had been doing this our entire marriage. He's been expending all of his sexual energy toward "fantasy objects." Let me tell you, this hurt as bad as if I had just found out my husband had been having a physical affair with someone else. It is such a betrayal and such a massive breach of trust.

Even if you don't intentionally access porn sites, you may get unsolicited e-mail about porn, sex, Viagra prescriptions, increasing penis size and hardness, available singles, foreign brides, and exciting new sex positions. As of this writing, if you Google the word *sex*, there are 440 *million* results. Google the word *porn*, and there are almost 96 million results. You don't have to be an Internet techie to find your way to sexually laden content, but you have to be a genius to avoid it.

Your husband may not be such a genius. He may be chatting online with women, spending money to view online pornography, uploading or downloading sexually explicit photos, having cybersex, or using the Internet to meet women. How can you tell if this is happening? Here are some telltale signs that your husband may be involved with cyberspace sexual options (and typically these behaviors increase over time):

- Spends long hours at his computer
- Seems secretive when he's online
- Abruptly changes what he's viewing when you walk into the room
- Gets agitated about not being able to get online or check e-mail
- Has secret e-mail accounts
- Has unexplained credit card expenses
- Keeps late hours to be at his computer
- Lies about the amount of time he spends online

And the Internet isn't the only sexual distraction; men still get offtrack the old-fashioned way, with magazines and photos. The end result is still the same.

So my husband says that he "just doesn't have the desire to have sex or be physical." Yet I have found girlie magazines hidden in his dresser drawer, porn movies he's rented when he thought I wasn't going to be home, pictures on the computer, AND pictures of my girlfriends from a bachelorette party in his dresser drawer. So, does he really not have a desire for sex? I think it means he does have a desire for sex. Maybe his sexual energy is directed to anything but me.

So what should you do if you find that your husband is siphoning off his sexual energy by engaging in destructive, compulsive sexual behaviors or cyberactivities that make you uncomfortable?

First of all, don't waste too much time or effort collecting evidence of your husband's activities. If you are troubled by his behavior an honest approach is best. You need to tell him about your concerns in a nonblaming way, using I-messages (you should be a pro at this by now). Describe the behavior that is troubling you, and explain the reasons for your discomfort. As always, make sure you're talking in action-oriented terms. For instance, tell him, "When you consistently stay online until 2:00 A.M. and you seem really uneasy when I'm in the computer room, I'm worried that you are doing something that may be hurtful to our marriage. I am really scared that you might be having an inappropriate relationship." Or, "It seems that every evening you go into the guest bedroom and turn on pornographic videos instead of having sex with me. That really hurts my feelings and worries me about the future of our marriage."

Now it's your husband's turn to respond. He can admit that you're right, deny your accusation entirely, or acknowledge that there's some truth to your suspicion but that you're making a much bigger deal out of it than need be. Now the ball is in your court. How should you respond?

If your husband admits there's a problem, and let's hope he does, then you should give him an opportunity to share with you anything he wants to say about his experiences. Really allow him to open up. Talk more about your feelings in a nonaccusatory way. Let this be an opportunity for him to come clean and for the two of you to decide to approach this issue as a team. See if you can get him to agree to cut back substantially on his online hours and devise a concrete plan for him to offer you further evidence that he is changing his ways. Let him know that you feel certain that your relationship will improve as he replaces his Internet activities or masturbatory behavior with quality time with you. Thank him for his honesty and ask that he schedule another time several weeks down the road for you to assess the progress you've both made.

If he admits that he has been engaging in behavior that concerns you but says it's not really a problem, you're halfway there. He might try to convince you that in some way, his current activities prevent him from engaging in behavior that would truly threaten your marriage. For instance, he might say that when he chats online, he's not meeting or having sex with anyone in person. He may also accuse you of overreacting or trying to micromanage him. After listening to his objection, you have to listen to your inner voice as to whether his behavior needs to stop. You may decide after hearing his perspective that he's right; it's no big deal. Or you may be thinking, "Nice try. It ain't gonna fly. This still is a big problem for me." In either case, trust yourself. You are the expert on you. Intimate online chatting and cybersex have all the characteristics of real-life affairs—secrecy, intimacy, and sexual fulfillment. That's why, no matter what your spouse tells you, his behavior feels like a betrayal. You're not crazy if you feel that way.

Rather than debate who's right or who's wrong, you need to take a firm stand. Tell him that he may be right in how he sees things, but as far as you're concerned, his behavior *feels* like betrayal or as if it is destructive to your marriage. You might consider giving him an article to read that bolsters your point of view. Insist that he do something to take your feelings into account. Then tell him in a solution-oriented way what it is that you would like him to change. It's important that you are realistic about your request so he doesn't feel overwhelmed and reject your suggestions flatout. For example, even if you are concerned about your husband's masturbation, it may be unrealistic to tell him to stop masturbating completely. Ask him to make more of an effort to connect with you sexually and use masturbation less as a sexual outlet. If your husband is willing to consider your feelings and do as you request, you're moving in the right direction.

What happens if your husband denies your allegations? This is a tough one. And I know that you'll be tempted to spend days, weeks, or months proving him wrong, but I suggest you not do that because it's enormously enervating and personally hurtful. If you feel convinced that he's been involved in sexual activity online or some other kind of sexual behavior that's unacceptable to you, talk with him about the negative changes you've observed in your marriage and your sexual relationship. Share what's been missing in your marriage and what you'd like to see changed. If your husband is willing to invest time and energy in making things better between you, it will make it impossible for him to continue his participation in extramarital activities. After all, you can't be in two places at the same time.

If, when your husband agrees to make changes, you doubt his sincerity, do yourself a favor and don't say anything. You need to give him the benefit of the doubt. He may be looking for a way to make life changes, but he might also want to save face. You need to let time pass and see what happens. If he stands by his word, great. If not, here are some alternatives women in my practice have used successfully.

The first suggestion is that you wait a while, and then revisit your conversation. Let him know that he hasn't done what he's told you he would do and share your disappointment. Ask for his suggestions about what to do next. If this leads to a productive conversation, you've made progress. If not or if he hasn't agreed to doing what you ask, I have another suggestion: if you can't lick 'em, join 'em. I've worked with many spouses who decide that they are going to show some curiosity in what their spouse finds so appealing. Rather than put the kibosh on your husband's interest in online pornography (or whatever behavior you're addressing), ask if you can join in! Promise that you will not get upset or be condemning; you just want to know more about what turns him on. If he agrees, go for it. You will see the kinds of things he's doing firsthand. You may discover that what's happening isn't as upsetting as you thought it might be. If it is, you will have more information to guide you in your next decision about your marriage. You might even find it exciting. In any case, including you removes the illicit or secretive nature of his actions, thereby possibly diffusing the erotic charge.

If your husband is really into Internet seduction, seduce him online! E-mail him with a hot, racy message. Get graphic. Become his cyberbabe. Going with the flow often works.

Remember the "do something different" strategy I've discussed repeatedly in this book? If what you're doing isn't working, do something different. If your husband knows that no matter how long he remains online, you will be waiting around for him to shut down his laptop so you can climb into his lap, make yourself less available to your husband when he graces you with his presence. If you've got kids, get a babysitter, and go out with your friends. Let him miss you. Even if you stay home, don't be at his beck and call. Make him realize that his offline life is changing.

When women confront their husbands with hard and fast evidence, sometimes that becomes the positive turning point in their marriage because the problem can be addressed openly and honestly for the first time.

> Michele, I just want you to know that my husband and I are now doing much better because I confronted him about online behavior . . . and since then, we have determined my husband has an issue with the whore/madonna complex. We are now finding ways to work with this issue . . . and around it. Suffice it to say, we are doing better now that his "secret" is out.

In other marriages, it doesn't quite work that way. Some husbands believe that the best defense is a good offense and become angry about their privacy being infringed on. They accuse their wives of spying and refuse to take any responsibility for their actions. If this happens, consult Chapter 11, "When He Resists."

INFIDELITY

If you suspect that the reason your husband has been less than sexual with you is that he's been having an affair, it stands to reason that you would be devastated. After all, there is this belief that men stray when their wives don't satisfy their sexual needs. But here you are, ready, willing, and able, and your husband is going outside your marriage for sex. What could be more hurtful?

How do you know if your husband is fooling around? Some of the telltale signs are very similar to the things he would do if he is involved with sexual activities on the Internet (page 189). Reread those tips and add them to these:

- Changes in his appearance or the way he dresses
- A new interest in working out
- Unexplained absences from work or home
- Secrecy about his cell phone or cell phone charges
- Secrecy about credit card bills

- Difficulty making eye contact or extreme defensiveness when you question him
- Overnight travel that seems out of the ordinary
- Unusual scents on his clothes
- A pervasive sense of distraction
- Unwillingness to include you in his activities

If you believe that your husband is having an affair, basically you should follow the exact same advice I offered in terms of confronting your husband about Internet activity. But for the sake of discussion, I am going to assume that you've gone beyond the suspicion stage and have discovered that your husband is in fact having an affair. Now what?

First, if you just learned of your husband's infidelity, I am certain that you don't know which end is up because you feel traumatized. Here you are, telling your husband that you miss him, you want him, you need to be closer sexually, and he's giving himself to someone else! That has got to be horrifically painful.

If you find yourself crying a lot, having trouble eating, overeating, experiencing sleeplessness, feeling anxious or depressed, or not being able to concentrate or function in your daily life, just know that all of these feelings are perfectly normal. You're not going crazy or "losing it." You're just a caring, loving person who has been betrayed and that's crazy-making. Don't be too hard on yourself. You need to take one day at a time. You won't be feeling as if you're drowning forever. I promise you.

You are probably desperate for answers about how the affair could have happened and how your spouse—the person you thought you could trust—could betray you. You wonder how he could look you straight in the face during all those discussions about his waning sex drive and lie repeatedly. You undoubtedly feel so disillusioned that you might even be questioning your own commitment to your marriage.

Although I completely understand why you might be thinking about leaving your husband, you need to know that many marriages survive infidelity. In fact, once couples do the work necessary to heal from the betrayal, their marriages can grow stronger than ever before. Don't allow your feelings of shock and devastation to prompt you to pack your bags immediately. Take a deep breath, make a plan, work the plan, and then decide on the future of your marriage. It might help to know that most affairs end after six months. This may not be true for your husband, but chances are that he will soon realize that the grass really isn't any greener on the other side.

If you have talked with your friends and relatives about your husband's bad choices, it's possible that they will be judgmental and urge you to leave your marriage. They are trying to protect you because they love you and don't want to see you hurt. But they don't live in your shoes; they're not you. Don't be too quick to take their advice. Divorce isn't the panacea many people think it is, particularly if you have kids. Since recovering from infidelity is a doable but challenging process, you may need more help than you receive from reading this section. The resources in Chapter 13 will direct you to other books you can read on the topic. You may also decide that you need professional help. In the meantime, here are some ways to start getting things on track.

Confront your husband with the information you have about his behavior. He will either own up to your accusation or deny it. If he owns up to it, he may be remorseful and wanting to make things right with you. Or he may acknowledge it, but tell you that he's not willing to stop his affair. Or he could deny it completely. I will explore each of these scenarios with you. You can skim through the material that does not apply to your situation and jump to the parts that may be more relevant.

He 'Fesses Up and Is Remorseful

Let's assume that you followed my suggestions in the earlier part of this chapter about discussing your concerns about infidelity and your husband took a deep breath and said, "You're right; I admit it. I'm having an affair." Then he tells you that he's sorry, he's been feeling really guilty, and he wants to get things back on track. He's worried about your reaction and about your marriage. As tough as his confession might be, this is the best of all possible worlds. Healing from infidelity is never easy, but the first step requires the betrayer to be honest. If your husband has been willing to do this, this is a really good thing, even if it hurts you. Recovery from this sort of betrayal takes a lot of time; although everyone is different, sometimes it takes months or years. You will need to be patient with yourself. Just when you think you're feeling better and have gotten a handle on this situation, something will remind you about the affair, and you will go tumbling down. People in my practice describe the feeling of being on a roller coaster: one day they're up, and the next day they're whirling in a downward spiral. When you descend, you will think that nothing has changed, that you'll always feel miserable, and that saving your marriage is an impossible feat. All people—even those who end up having wonderful marriages—feel that way.

If you're up to the task of rebuilding your marriage and reclaiming your sex life, here are the steps you need to take:

- **Give yourself permission to feel a whole range of emotional responses.**

The emotions you will experience as you go through this process will make PMS seem like child's play. You might feel everything from intense rage to disbelief, hurt, devastation, disillusionment, and debilitating sadness. Then as soon as you get a grip on one emotion, another will take its place. Fasten your seat belt; you're just along for the ride. Don't try to deny, avoid, or purge yourself of these feelings. They'll simply hang around longer that way. Just notice, acknowledge, and honor them. It's part of what makes you human.

- **Express your feelings, and ask questions about the affair if you so desire.**

Many people, especially women, are curious about the affair. Research tells us that if the betrayed person has questions, she must be permitted to have those questions answered for healing to begin. I wholeheartedly agree. If you want some of the details of what happened and why it happened, your husband should agree to scheduling conversations with you to clear the air. He needs to be honest with his responses and patient with you. If he resists, you may need some professional help to get you past this hump. If he seems resistant, it's not because he doesn't love you or care about your feelings. It's probably that he feels so uncomfortable, so full of shame that it's hard to him to deal directly with his poor decisions. Make it clear that this is a necessary—and temporary—part of the process you need to go through.

If your husband is willing to share information with you, you need to listen without attacking him, because otherwise he will defend himself, and that is not a good thing. Just listen, ask for clarification, talk calmly about your feelings, and let him elaborate. You also have to check into yourself and see whether having the facts is helpful or hurtful. If it is helpful, keep doing it until the need to do so subsides. It will eventually. If his information leaves you feeling worse, then no matter how curious you might be, you should reconsider asking those kinds of questions.

The bottom line here is that you must be in the driver's seat in terms of making the decision about what's talked about. You've been betrayed, and your husband needs to do the lion's share of the work to win back your trust. You deserve this.

• *Spend extra time together.*

If you recently discovered that your husband has been unfaithful, it will help if you can spend extra time together. Most people find this soothing and reassuring. This means that you and your husband might temporarily have to adjust your normal working schedules so that you can be in each other's presence. Don't use this time together as an opportunity to constantly discuss the affair. Use it to do something together that feels comforting and connecting. You will have a time to talk about the infidelity, but you also need a time when you're not talking about it.

• *You are entitled to know your husband's whereabouts at all times.*

While you're rebuilding trust, it's important that your husband agrees to fill you in on his whereabouts. That means you get to know his schedule and, if you find it comforting, that he calls you when you're apart just to touch base. The more he can reassure you that he really is where he says he's going to be, the more quickly you will work through this process. If your husband tells you that by making himself accountable to you in this way makes him feel like a child, remind him that this level of reassurance is only temporary. When people go through a crisis period, they often have to do things they ordinarily don't have to do until they get through it. This is the case right now. Your husband doesn't have to like the fact that he's reporting to you about his day; he just has to do it. It's an act of real giving.

• *Ask for reassurances.*

If you need reassurance about your husband's whereabouts or his feelings, ask rather than accuse. I've worked with many women whose husbands have been unfaithful, and when these men arrive home for dinner ten minutes late, their wives light into them. They say, "Where were you? I bet you were on your cell with her. Or did you go to her house? What were you doing? Why the hell are you late?" How do *you* think you would respond to that?

There are very real reasons that you will be feeling insecure. It goes with the territory, and you absolutely deserve to be reassured. However, *loving* reassurance is what you're after, and you have to ask for it in a way that will make getting it more likely. Simply say, "I know it was probably nothing, but when you came home late from work, it really scared me. I started to wonder whether you stopped by to see her. I hate feeling this way, so help me with it, please. Tell me why you were late." That statement is more likely to encourage your husband to give you the love you deserve.

• *Discuss why the affair happened.*

Infidelity is not always a sign of a troubled marriage. It may just be that your husband had a lapse in judgment. But it really behooves you to look into the matter more deeply. Your husband may or may not know why he did what he did, but you should discuss it nonetheless. If there are underlying issues in your marriage, you will want to address them, which also will make the bond in your marriage stronger.

This is not to say that if you and your husband were having relationship problems prior to his straying, these problems *caused* your husband to go outside your marriage. He made his choices all by himself. However, the more information you have about his feelings, the better armed you are to together make your marriage a happier place to be.

Men stray for all sorts of reasons. Some men have affairs to meet sexual needs. Although you picked up this book because you have been longing for more sex with your husband, you need to ask yourself whether there was a time in your marriage, perhaps for long periods, when you consistently turned him down. Could it be that his ego got bruised, and he began looking for sexual satisfaction outside your marriage? Or could he be bored and be looking outside your marriage for sexual novelty?

Some men feel taken for granted, and an affair helps them feel special and more appreciated. Some men stray because they feel criticized by their wives and adored by their affair partners. Some men have affairs as a cry for help. They may have made some attempt to tell their wives about their unhappiness in their marriages but to no avail. The discovery of an affair becomes an opportunity to deal with the problems in the relationship. Out of desperation to save their marriages, the wives were more open to hearing their husbands' concerns.

And last, but not least, are the people who have affairs because of a sexual addiction. Men with sexual addictions often have sound marriages and love their wife, but have a seemingly insatiable need to engage in certain sexual behaviors, even if it means hurting those closest to them. Unless the addicted person acknowledges the problem and gets professional help to understand himself and learn impulse control, there is little his wife can do to end the sexual escapades.

- **Ask whether there are things he would like to change about your marriage.**

This might be difficult for you if you're thinking, "Who gives a damn about what *he* thinks? *I'm* the one who's hurt!" And it makes sense for you to feel that way. However, identifying the weak spots in your marriage gives you and your spouse the opportunity to work on them together as a team. He will feel happier and more committed to you, and when that happens, you'll feel happier too. Remember that the goal is to stabilize your marriage, rebuild trust, and find new ways to connect intimately.

- **Forgive.**

There is no question that your marriage won't thrive unless you eventually forgive your husband. Unless you forgive, you won't feel joy or closeness. This is one of the hardest steps in the recovery process, but you can't forgive blindly. In order for you to truly let go of the past, your husband has a job to do: He has to win back your trust. He has to be willing to do whatever it takes to ease your mind, heart, and soul.

In addition to the responsibilities that I already mentioned, your husband needs to end the affair. He needs to do some soul searching to determine why he gave himself permission to stray. He needs to feel and demonstrate genuine remorse. He needs to help you feel that he understands how badly you've been hurt by his choices. He needs to promise—and mean it—that he will *never* stray from your marriage again and that he will change his life in such a way to eliminate unnecessary temptations. This might mean changing jobs, schedules, or avoiding dinners out with colleagues, for example.

As you go through this process, your husband will want you to speed up your recovery. From time to time, he might feel impatient with your lingering mistrust, sadness, or anxiety about the future. But regardless of his feelings, he needs to be patient and loving with you. He needs to show you that he will be there for you even when you continue to struggle with confusing emotions.

Once your husband goes the extra mile to help you heal, forgiveness will come more easily to you. You will find that your negative feelings about the past will begin to fade, and you will realize that while forgiving takes strength, the fortitude required to forgive pales in comparison to the energy it takes to hold a grudge. Just keep in mind that forgiveness isn't a feeling that comes and goes; it's a decision. You must *decide* that you are going to start over with a clean slate. You won't forget the past; you will learn from it. And you can both make tomorrow better.

He 'Fesses Up and Won't Quit His Affair or Denies Any Wrongdoing

I am thirty-one years old, and I can't believe what has happened in my marriage. I've been begging my husband for more physical affection. We have been married for three years, and out of the blue, he just stopped having sex with me. He had been such a good lover before, so I started to wonder if he was seeing someone else. I looked at his cell phone bills and found a number that he calls all the time, even late at night. I told him that I know what's going on, and he admitted it. I cried a lot and told him he had to quit calling her, but he said that he might love her and he's not going to stop seeing her yet.

My parents know about the situation, and so do my close girlfriends. Everyone wants me to leave. My parents want me to come home to them. But we have a son together, and I still love him, even if he's being a jerk. I know this sounds stupid, but I still want my marriage back. I'm willing to forgive and forget if he will just agree to work on our relationship. Am I being ridiculous, or does this make sense?

Perhaps your husband admits he's involved with someone, but he isn't willing to cut off the relationship. Then what do you do? You might be tempted to leave, but remember that most affairs end once the bloom is off the rose. If, despite your husband's choice, you decide to fight for your marriage, I have a few suggestions.

First, know that you will be battling your own pride because that little inner voice will keep wondering why in the world you're staying in a sexless, seemingly loveless marriage. If your marriage were to continue in this vein, there would be no reason to stay. However, I've seen many marriages transform once the unfaithful partner comes back to planet earth. So if you want to wait things out and stack the deck in the favor of your marriage in the meantime, there are some things you can do:

- **Stop pushing, pleading, or chasing.**

Once you discover that your husband has been unfaithful, it's normal for you to want to get him to give up that relationship. You might try to reason with your spouse, and if that doesn't work, you might beg, plead, or cry. When people fear losing someone or something, it's normal to try to hold on more tightly. Unfortunately, the more you press him, the more your husband will want to pull away. If you continue pursuing him, you might push him into the arms of the other woman permanently.

No matter how hard it might be, you need to stop yourself from trying to convince your husband to end his affair; your requests or demands will only make him more determined to follow his bliss. If you want to save your marriage, you need to back off. This will probably be the hardest thing you've ever done in your life, but you have to give him some breathing room for a while. He has to get to the point where working on your marriage is *his* idea, not yours.

- **Stop talking about the affair.**

When a husband willingly ends an affair, it's okay to talk about the affair as much as necessary to heal from the pain. This does not apply to you if your husband consciously decides to continue his extramarital relationship. Since he's not yet ready to change, if you talk about the affair, he will view it as nagging. Nagging will make him want to avoid being with you. Again, this will be very challenging for you to do. But for the time being, it's a necessary step in trying to get things back on track.

• Don't ask about the status of your marriage.

I know you will have all sorts of questions about your marriage and where you stand, but now's not the time to ask them. He's very confused at the moment, and if you press him for answers, you won't like what you hear. Along these lines, don't keep telling your husband you love him. Since he's not certain about his feelings about the marriage, he can't reciprocate every time he hears your professions of love. In fact, when you say, "I love you," it's a reminder that he might not feel the same way, and you don't want to remind him of this. Keep your feelings to yourself.

• Be more upbeat.

Although you're probably not feeling so great right now, if you're down in the dumps in his presence, you will not be too enticing to be around; imagine how that will compare to the other woman. So when he's around, act as if you're feeling confident that everything is going to be fine. Show him that even if your marriage doesn't survive what's happening, *you're* going to be okay. In fact, you're going to be even more than okay. You'll be *great!* Be the person he loved when he met you, and you will remind him of why you married in the first place.

One more thing: being perkier will be challenging. Perhaps you will deserve an Academy Award. But the more you act as if you're doing okay, the more you will start feeling okay. It works that way.

• Do some investigative work.

When I say *investigative work*, I don't mean that you should snoop around to find out more details about his philandering. What you should try to figure out is what is so fascinating about the other woman. It might help you understand what your husband feels is missing in your marriage. Here are some things to think about.

Does she flatter him a great deal, building his ego? Is she spontaneous, willing to do things at the spur of the moment when you like to have things planned months in advance? Is she a good listener, always interested in what he has to say? You need to find out what need your spouse is fulfilling by spending time with this person so that you can do a better job fulfilling that need yourself.

• **Take care of yourself.**

Until your husband comes to his senses, you need to take good care of yourself. Do things that help you keep your sanity—things that you enjoy. Go places with your kids. Spend time with friends. Go on a vacation if you can. Start a new hobby. Exercise regularly. Go to a spa. Keep a journal, noting your triumphs and your strengths. Visit my Web site, www.divorce busting.com, for other ideas and lots of support from the online community.

If things go as planned, your husband in time will see the new you, and he'll start to realize that you're the person he wants in his life. Even so, it will take time to rebuild your sexual relationship. For one thing, you should be concerned about health issues. If he's interested in being sexual with you, you should ask that he first be tested for sexually transmitted diseases.

Even if you've been successful in getting him to terminate his affair, don't expect that you will always feel ecstatic. Feelings of resentment and anger that you've staved off for so long might bubble to the surface. If so, this is normal. Once your husband has decided to return and has agreed to work on your marriage, I strongly suggest that you both seek marital therapy to work through the hard issues ahead of you. And naturally, rebuilding your sexual relationship remains a top priority.

If despite your sticking to the outlined plan, your husband continues his affair, it may be time to shift gears. Before you decide to end your marriage, here's an approach worth trying, but don't do this unless you're truly fed up and ready to call it quits: tell him that you love him enough to let him go. Tell him that you don't want to live like this anymore. Draw a line in the sand. Don't waffle. Tell him that unless he ends his affair, your marriage is over. Then back off completely. Don't initiate conversation. Don't spend time with him. Don't sit in the same room. Make sure your schedules don't coincide. Be brief in your responses to him. If you have children, limit your interactions to things that concern them. Continue this emotional cutoff until you feel certain that the affair has ended. The burden of proof now becomes his. Let him do the work. If he shows interest in winning you back, let him know that you are skeptical. Make him believe that he has one, and only one, chance to regain your trust. Make him work for your attention.

This technique will force you to really stand up for yourself, and it will take courage. Once you give him the ultimatum, you have to be willing to stand your ground. If you don't mean it, he will sense it. So, as I said before, don't pull out the big guns unless you're willing to fire. I hope you won't have to do that. However, if you're convinced that he's cheating and after working on it for a while, none of the strategies seem to make a difference, I recommend that you read my book, *The Divorce Remedy*, or speak to a Divorce Busting Coach to sort out what to do next.

SEXUAL IDENTITY CONFUSION

Sometimes men lose interest in sex with their wives because they discover that they are gay. This happens much more frequently than people think. Many gay men are married with children. How does this happen?

There is a great deal of pressure in our culture to be straight, and people often try to mold their lives to fit in. They repress their sexuality and deny their attraction to people of the same sex. They want to be "normal," so they date, marry, and have children. Men often believe that when they marry, their homosexual feelings will go away. Marriage will "fix" them.

But eventually, their feelings of attraction for other men become overwhelming. They recognize that their sexual fantasies are often about other men, and they find themselves longing for a relationship with a man. At some point, they must admit to themselves that although they love their wives and their children, their desire for a same-sex relationship can no longer be ignored.

When men finally decide to come out of the closet, although it may be freeing to ascend from darkness, it is often truly devastating to them, their wives, and their families. Many of these marriages have lasted for decades, and there rarely are simple solutions to this dilemma.

Do you think that one of the reasons your husband has limited interest in sex with you may be because he's gay but hasn't come out of the closet? If so, here are some things to consider.

First, make sure you aren't assuming your husband is gay simply because he's not interested in you sexually. This book is filled with reasons a man might lose interest; being gay is only one of many. Second, don't jump to conclusions that your husband is gay if his temperament or personality isn't mucho macho. Women tell me that they're worried their husbands are gay when their men have stereotypical female characteristics such as being sensitive, emotional, artistic, gentle, and laid back or are sports averse. Not all men resemble the Marlborough Man image; there is great diversity in the stuff that good men are made of. Some are much more metrosexual than others.

But what should you do if you suspect that your husband might be gay or bisexual and struggling with how to handle the truth about himself? Here is some great advice from Ramone Johnson, a gay expert on the Web site www.about.com. He suggests that when you're ready, you ask your husband about his sexuality and sexual history:

- Pick a time when you both can be alone.
- Let him know you are concerned about his current behavior (for example, talking in male chatrooms, hinting toward a sexual attraction to men) and that you suspect he may be gay or bisexual. He may get angry or defensive, so assure him that you are asking because you care and deserve his honesty.
- Ask him if he's ever been with other men or has a desire to be with them.
- Inquire about his sexual history. Even if you already know, ask again with detailed questions.
- Tell him you would like to practice safe sex from this point on for your own protection.

If your husband admits to having homosexual or bisexual feelings, you need to know that it is not, let me say this again, *not* a reflection on you or your inadequacies as a woman. We can't help whom we're attracted to. In the same way that you're attracted to men not by decision but by nature's call, your husband is attracted to men. It doesn't mean that you've failed in any way. It just is.

If your husband comes out of the closet, this will be a very tough time for you, especially if you have had little or no clue about his inclination. Getting professional advice can help you decide what to do next. Learning that your husband is gay may not be acceptable to you, and you may decide to leave your marriage. If this is your choice—and only you know the right path to take—you can still learn how to part amicably and remain friends. Divorce in and of itself can be devastating; hostile divorce is traumatic and debilitating, especially for the children. Check out resources for mediators in your area who can help you dissolve your marriage without contempt or unnecessary litigation.

However, before you jump to any conclusions about the future of your marriage, you need to know that there are many couples who have decided to stay together for lots of reasons—they love each other, they love the family, they have financial reasons, or they're simply great friends. They choose to make peace with each other and accept who they are. Rather than focus on what's missing in the marriage, these folks make a conscious decision to focus on the positive aspects of their lives together. They love each other, they're good teammates, and sex has never been the fundamental reason they've stayed together. Their marriage is a happy one, albeit less than perfect. But when you come down to it, who's marriage is perfect?

If you decide to stay in your marriage, you will need some help in figuring out how to satisfy yourself sexually and deal with other difficult issues that will inevitably arise. When you get help, make sure you talk with someone who will support your decision to stay. Many therapists will not understand. That's because situations like yours, although somewhat common, are commonly not discussed, and many professionals simply don't recognize or support nontraditional choices. Again, if you can't find a marriage-friendly therapist in your area, Divorce Busting telephone coaches can help you sort through these issues (see Chapter 13 for the phone number).

~IV~

More to Come

~

CHAPTER THIRTEEN

Additional Resources

Our journey together is coming to an end. It is my sincerest hope that you have found comfort and direction in my words. I also hope that I have helped you to feel less alone and better equipped to tackle whatever relationship challenges still lie before you. Marriage is never easy. I'm certain you know this firsthand. Even if you've been able to improve your sexual relationship in big ways, you can depend on the fact that your marriage-enhancing job is not over. It never is. Marriage is a work in progress. Just ask people who have been married for many years. They'll tell you the truth about long-term relationships. It is said that "we connect through our similarities. It is through our differences that we grow." And, boy, that's the truth.

So whether your sexual relationship is exactly where you want it to be right now—and I sincerely hope that's the case—or it still is in need of some repair, just know that this experience—this challenge to create more love, connection, sexuality, sensuality, and affection—has made you the incredible person you are: a woman who fights for what's important in life and love. That's you. You're courageous and strong. I know that all those around you benefit from your wisdom. Thank you for letting me walk this path with you and entrusting me with your marriage.

And because you know that touch is so important, feel free to stay in touch. Drop me a line at Michele@DivorceBusting.com.

There are many wonderful resources available, and I want to make sure that you have them at your fingertips. Here they are.

RESOURCES

The Divorce Busting Center. Michele Weiner Davis is the founder. If you'd like to follow up on the ideas in *The Sex-Starved Wife*, we provide telephone coaching for couples dealing with sexual and other relationship issues. Michele and her staff are dedicated to helping couples work things out rather than get out of their marriages. For a complete description of services provided, visit divorcebusting.com or sexstarvedwife.com. You can also call 800-664-2435 or 303-444-7004.

AASECT-The American Association of Sexuality Educators, Counselors and Therapists. If you are in search of a licensed sex therapist, your best bet is to contact AASECT. You can visit the Web site at www.aasect.org or call headquarters at 804-752-0026.

RECOMMENDED READING

Body Image
Andersen, A., L. Cohn, and L. Holbrook. *Making Weight: Healing Men's Conflicts with Food, Weight, and Shape.* Carlsbad, Calif.: Gurze Books, 2000. Written for both men and their families, this book addresses men's concerns about physical appearance, attractiveness, and eating disorders.

Krasnow, M. *My Life as a Male Anorexic.* Binghamton, NY: Haworth Press, 1996. A memoir that dispels any myths that only women suffer eating disorders.

Pope Jr., H. G., K. A. Phillips, and R. Olivardia. *The Adonis Complex: The Secret Crisis of Male Body Obsession.* New York: Free Press, 2000. Exposes the truth around many men's preoccupation with body image.

Depression and Mid-life Issues
Conway, J. *Men in Midlife Crisis.* Rev. ed. Colorado Springs: Chariot Victor Publishing, 1997. Suggestions and advice for all men going through midlife crisis on how to avoid unnecessary consequences such as divorce or job loss.

Diamond, J. *The Irritable Male Syndrome: Understanding and Managing the Four Key Causes of Depression and Aggression.* New York: Rodale Books, 2005. Written for men and the women who love them. An exploration of the transitional moods and changes, fluctuating testosterone levels, biochemical imbalances, and loss of masculine identity that offers different treatment options.

Real, T. *I Don't Want to Talk About It: Overcoming the Secret Legacy of Male Depression.* New York: Scribner, 1998. Written by a prominent marriage counselor who uncovers the secrets about male depression, etiology, and treatment.

Sheffield, A. *Depression Fallout: The Impact of Depression on Couples and What You Can Do to Preserve the Bond.* New York: HarperCollins, 2003. Focuses on the spouses and families of the depressed person and outlines what the author calls the "five stages of depression fallout." Provides hope for coping with and understanding the depressed spouse (www.depressionfallout.com).

Relationships and Intimacy

Barbach, L. *For Each Other: Sharing Sexual Intimacy.* New York: Signet, 2001. Exercises and practices that help deal with the different facets of sex, including physical and psychological.

Haltzman, S. *The Secrets of Happily Married Women.* San Francisco: Jossey-Bass, 2008. "Learn to communicate more about the connection you seek so your husband really knows what it looks like and how to do it."

Hendrix, H. *Getting the Love You Want.* New York: Henry Holt & Co., 1988. This book helps couples become aware of how childhood experiences impact their marriages and offers ways to achieve intimacy.

Love, P. *The Truth About Love: The Highs, the Lows, and How You Can Make It Last Forever.* New York: Fireside, 2001. Straight-shooting advice about the realities of love.

Love, P., and S. Stosny. *How to Improve Your Marriage Without Talking About it: Finding Love Beyond Words.* New York: Broadway Books, 2007. An innovative book by two great writers and presenters that teaches couples how to communicate through action rather than rely solely on words.

Sheehy, G. *Understanding Men's Passages: Discovering the New Map of Men's Lives.* New York: Random House, 1999. Explores the fears and secrets of men that they are afraid to discuss with one another and the women in their lives, including waning sexual potency and male menopause.

Weiner-Davis, M. *Getting Through to the Man You Love: The No-Nonsense, No-Nagging Guide for Women.* New York: Golden Books, 1999. Teaches women strategies for reaching their husbands and creating relationship change. Entertaining and educational.

Weiner-Davis, M. *Divorce Remedy: Proven 7-Step Program for Saving Your Marriage.* New York: Simon & Schuster, 2001. A practical program to help couples get their marriages back on track even if one spouse has half a foot out the door.

Romance and Fun

Corn, L. *101 Nights of Grrreat Romance: Secret Sealed Seductions for Fun-Loving Couples.* Oklahoma City: Park Avenue Publishers, 1996. Sealed plans for a night of romance and seduction, with scenarios and specific suggestions for a great evening. They cannot be read until they are torn out, and couples take turns surprising each other.

Godek, G. J. *Love Coupons.* Naperville, Ill.: Sourcebooks. 1997. Forty-four ways to enhance your relationship in simple and fun ways.

Schwartz, P., and J. Lever. *The Great Sex Weekend: A 48-Hour Guide to Rekindling Sparks for Bold, Busy, or Bored Lovers.* New York: Perigee Trade, 2000. A weekend guide to breaking old patterns of boredom and tedium in the bedroom.

Webb, M. *The Romantic's Guide: Hundreds of Creative Tips for a Lifetime of Love.* New York: Hyperion, 2000. For couples who are looking for creative and new ideas to keep romance in their lives.

Sensuality and Spirituality

Deida, D. *Dear Lover: A Woman's Guide to Men, Sex, and Love's Deepest Bliss.* Louisville, KY.: Sounds True, 2005. A man's perspective of what works for men—their wants and needs.

Deida, D. *The Way of the Superior Man: A Spiritual Guide to Mastering the Challenges of Woman, Work, and Sexual Desire.* Louisville, KY.: Sounds True, 2004. A book written by a man for other men who are interested in experiencing a rich and deep relationship with the woman in their life.

Kuriansky, J. *The Complete Idiot's Guide to Tantric Sex.* 2nd ed. New York: Alpha, 2004. A description of every aspect of this ancient sexual practice. The book includes Tantric sex therapy techniques and tips, as well as a listing of national Tantra instructors and workshops.

Ogden, G. *The Heart and Soul of Sex: Making the ISIS Connection.* Boston: Trumpeter, 2006. Based on a landmark sex survey, Integrating Sexuality and Spirituality (ISIS), sex therapist Ogden writes this book for women, encouraging them to go beyond sexual performance to an integration of self, spirituality, and enjoyment.

Richardson, D. *The Heart of Tantric Sex: A Unique Guide to Love and Sexual Fulfillment.* New ed. Berkeley, Calif.: O Books, 2003. A user-friendly guide to the basics of Tantric sex.

Sexual Addiction

Carnes, P. *Don't Call It Love: Recovery from Sexual Addiction.* Reprint ed. New York: Bantam, 1992. An outline by an expert on sexual addiction, of sexual addictions, their causes (including men who were sexually abused as children), and the path to recovery.

Carnes, P. *Out of the Shadows: Understanding Sexual Addiction.* 3rd ed. Center City, Minn.: Markham: Hazelden, 2001. Written by a pioneer in the treatment of male sexual addiction, including Internet porn addiction.

Maheu, M. M., and R. Subotnik. *Infidelity on the Internet: Virtual Relationships and Real Betrayal.* Naperville, Ill.: Sourcebooks, 2001. Explores the dangers and consequences of Internet infidelity and its impact on couples.

Sbraga, T. P., and W. T. O'Donohue. *The Sex Addiction Workbook: Proven Strategies to Help You Regain Control of Your Life.* Oakland, Calif.: New Harbinger Publications, 2004. Questionnaires for readers to assess their sexual problems and addictions with clear direction on how to overcome these problems to enjoy healthy and balanced lives.

Sexual Desire

Braverman, E. *Male Sexual Fitness.* New York: McGraw-Hill, 1999. A simple and inexpensive guide for men that contains questionnaires to help specify problem areas around issues of sexual desire and suggestions on naturally taking care of the male body to increase sexual libido.

Cervenka, K. *In the Mood, Again: A Couple's Guide to Reawakening Sexual Desire.* Oakland, Calif.: New Harbinger Publications, 2003. Rather than focusing on the male's or female's sexual shortcomings, this book looks at the couple's dynamic. Uses comfortable, fun, and easy exercises for couples to learn to communicate more effectively about and stimulate their sex life.

Fisch, H., and S. Braun. *The Male Biological Clock: The Startling News About Aging, Sexuality, and Fertility in Men.* New York: Free Press, 2004. Focuses on male infertility and goes into detail about the role of testosterone, erectile dysfunction, and the importance of proper diet and exercise as they relate to sexual problems.

Love, P., and J. Robinson. *Hot Monogamy: Essential Steps to More Passionate, Intimate Lovemaking.* Reprint ed. New York: Plume, 1995. A great book for couples wanting to boost sexual desire, build passion, and learn how to communicate about sex.

McCarthy, Barry. "Resilient Sexual Desire in Heterosexual Couples," *Family Journal,* vol. 14, no. 1 (2006), 59-64.

McCarthy, B. W., and E. J. McCarthy. *Rekindling Desire: A Step-by-Step Program to Help Low-Sex and No-Sex Marriages.* Oxford: Routledge, 2003. A ten-step program, aimed at both men and women suffering from low sexual desire, showing couples how to uncover their own issues that may be prohibiting sexual desire, such as shame, anger, or guilt. Also discusses medical side effects and physical sexual dysfunctions.

Perel, E. *Mating in Captivity: Reconciling the Erotic and the Domestic.* New York: HarperCollins, 2006. Does familiarity breed sexual boredom? Find out and learn what to do about it.

Stodart, R., J. Tomkiw, B. Tomkiw, and the Philip Lief Group. *Total Sex: Men's Fitness*

Magazine's Complete Guide to Everything Men Need to Know and Want to Know About Sex. New York: HarperCollins, 1999. Written specifically for men and covers everything from general anatomy, physiology, and male hormones to what men can expect sexually at different ages.

Weiner-Davis, M. *The Sex-Starved Marriage: Boosting Your Marriage Libido.* New York: Simon & Schuster, 2003. Written for both the high- and low-desire spouse to help them work as a team to boost the marriage libido.

Sexual Health for Men

Alterowitz, R., and B. Alterowitz. *Intimacy with Impotence: The Couple's Guide to Better Sex After Prostate Disease.* Cambridge, Mass.: Da Capo Press, 2004. A practical and informative guide written by a prostate cancer survivor and his wife. Provides information on commercial therapies and medications, as well as how to reestablish intimacy and sex despite impotency.

Birch, R. *Sex and the Aging Male: Understanding and Coping with Change.* Exp. ed. Rye, N.Y.: PEC Pub, 2001. A book intended for men age forty-five and older that takes a realistic look at the sexual consequences of aging and offers practical advice on how to stay sexually active.

Jones, S. J., and B. Dole. *Overcoming Impotence: A Leading Urologist Tells You Everything You Need to Know.* Amherst, Mass.: Prometheus Books, 2003. Focuses on erectile dysfunction, with reviews of a full range of treatment options and a look at new and promising drugs. Written in a lighthearted manner that will put many men at ease.

Laken, V., and K. Laken. *Making Love Again: Hope for Couples Facing Loss of Sexual Intimacy.* Westport, Conn.: Dialogue Press, 2002. Candid and practical help written for couples facing male sexual dysfunction due to diabetes, prostate cancer, injury, or psychological reasons.

Metz, M., and B. W. McCarthy. *Coping with Erectile Dysfunction: How to Regain Confidence and Enjoy Great Sex.* Oakland, Calif.: New Harbinger Publications, 2004. A couple-centered approach by two prominent sex therapists who offer a look at the social, biological, and psychological causes of erectile dysfunction and offer a treatment plan. The book suggests a cooperative process between the couple in tackling this problem.

Metz, M., and B. W. McCarthy. *Coping with Premature Ejaculation: How to Overcome PE, Please Your Partner and Have Great Sex.* Oakland, Calif.: New Harbinger Publications, 2004. Tackles the subject of male sexual performance and analyzes male sexual desire. A resource for couples that offers practical treatment strategies.

Milsten, R., and J. Slowinski. *The Sexual Male: Problems and Solutions.* New York: Norton, 2000. An informative and thorough male sex manual on male menopause, intimacy, and psychological factors. A self-evaluation section offers direction that helps men deal with actual or potential impotence.

Shippen, E., and W. Fryer. *The Testosterone Syndrome: The Critical Factor for Energy, Health, and Sexuality: Reversing the Male Menopause.* New York: M. Evans and Company, 2001. A discussion of the importance of testosterone and its correlation to a healthy sex life.

Spark, R. *Sexual Health for Men.* New York: Perseus Books Group, 2000. An explanation written by a distinguished endocrinologist and associate clinical professor of medicine at Harvard Medical School that explains the effects of drug and alcohol use on sexual function, as well as the role of male hormones.

Tan, R. *The Andropause Mystery: Unraveling Truths About the Male Menopause.* Houston: Amred Consulting, 2001. An informative book about male hormonal changes, including changes in the bedroom.

Zilbergeld, B. *The New Male Sexuality: The Truth about Men, Sex and Pleasure.* Rev. ed. New York: Bantam, 1999. Contains a section on resolving male sexual problems. The book is forthright, normalizing, and encouraging.

Talking About Sex

Joannides, P. *Guide to Getting It On!* Waldport, Ore.: Goofy Foot Press, 2006. A book for couples to read together (make it a date night) that can provide the reticent male the voice to be able to talk about sex. Informal and fun to read. Also offers tips, techniques, positions, photographs, and slang terms that will put its readers at ease.

Tannen, D. *You Just Don't Understand: Women and Men in Conversation.* New York: Harper Paperbacks, 2001. A classic book about the differences in gender communication. While not specifically focused on the subject of sex, the book offers an invaluable way for men and women to understand one another in conversation, negotiation, and understanding.

Techniques

Blue, V. *The Ultimate Guide to Fellatio: How to Go Down on a Man and Give Him Mind-Blowing Pleasure.* San Francisco: Cleis Press, 2002. A useful guide to the art of fellatio, with education about the male sexual cycle and male orgasm.

Kerner, I. *She Comes First: The Thinking Man's Guide to Pleasuring a Woman.* New York: Regan Books, 2004. Practical and candid advice to men with specific techniques to lead women to orgasm. An excellent resource for the man whose low sexual desire comes from feeling incompetent when it comes to pleasing his woman.

Kerner, I. *He Comes Next: The Thinking Woman's Guide to Pleasuring a Man.* New York: Regan Books, 2006. A companion book to *She Comes First, He Comes Next* offers women expert advice on understanding the nature of male desire and practical sex techniques that may be the missing key to his low sexual desire.

McCarthy, B. W., and E. J. McCarthy. *Male Sexual Awareness: Increasing Sexual Satisfaction*. Rev. and updated ed. New York: Carroll & Graf Publishers, 1998. Emphasizes to men the need to focus on pleasure rather than performance as well as the effects on sex and aging. Includes case studies.

Paget, L. *How to Be a Great Lover: Girlfriend-to-Girlfriend Totally Explicit Techniques That Will Blow His Mind*. New York: Broadway, 1999. An informal yet explicit guide to empower the woman to be part of taking more control in the bedroom.

Winks, C., and A. Semans. *The Good Vibrations Guide to Sex: The Most Complete Sex Manual Ever Written*. 3rd ed. San Francisco: Cleis Press; 2002. A sex manual that goes outside the boundaries of more traditional sex manuals, including fantasy, eroticism, and sex toys.

PRODUCTS AND SOURCES

www.bettersex.com. A Web site that offers a professional and user-friendly resource for couples to discover "ideas, information and products that make sex more fun and rewarding." Well known for the Better Sex Video Series, some of which include the recent Better Sex Video Series: Sexplorations (2005): Volume 1: *Advanced Sexual Techniques and Positions*, Volume 2: *Sex Secrets, Tips and Turn-Ons*, and Volume 3: *Erotic Sex Play and Beyond*. The Better Sex Advanced Techniques 2 Series has these volumes: Volume 1: *Sexual Positions for Lovers*, Volume 2: *Unlocking the Secrets of the G-Spot*, Volume 3: *10 Secrets to Great Sex*, and Volume 4: *Better Sex Guide to Enjoying Guilty Pleasures*.

www.evesgarden.com. A Web site whose motto is, "We grow pleasurable things for women." Available for purchase are helpful DVDs and videos, sex toys, audiotapes, games, magazines, and books. Confidentiality is always assured. Several products featured in *Oprah Magazine*.

www.goodvibrations.com. The Web site provides access to information, toys, books, an online magazine, videos, and DVDs to promote healthy attitudes about sex

www.sexuality.org. Frank information and discussions around sexuality and enhancing sexual pleasure. Educational DVDs, toys, and books offering basic sex tips are available for purchase.

MARRIAGE EDUCATION

www.divorcebusting.com for relation-building seminars

www.smartmarriages.com for information about seminars held nationally and internationally

Index